Husbandry, Medicine & Surgery in
CAPTIVE REPTILES

FREDRIC L. FRYE, D.V.M.

Veterinary Practitioner:
   Berkeley Dog & Cat Hospital
   Berkeley, California

Research Associate:
   Steinhart Aquarium
   Golden Gate Park
   San Francisco, California

   Donner Laboratory
   Lawrence Berkeley Laboratory
   Berkeley, California

Lecturer:
   University of California
   San Francisco and Davis

   University of California
   Extension Division, Berkeley

Photographs by the Author

 VM Publishing, Inc., 144 North Nettleton, Bonner Springs, Kansas 66012

1973

Library of Congress Catalog Card No. 73-77929

Dedicated to my wife **BRUCYE**

CONTENTS

Foreword

REPTILES, ranging from giant snakes and crocodilia down to diminutive lizards and snakes which can be easily cupped in a child's hand, have been kept captive by man since the beginning of recorded history. But this volume, devoted to captive reptiles, is the first work if its kind to be published!

Within this volume, Dr. Frye has set down, as a labor of love, some 20 years of personal experience and observations in ministering to reptiles.

Dr. Frye's efforts, professional and precise, but warm throughout with deep humanitarian concern for reptiles, will surely be a most valuable addition to the working knowledge of all those who are concerned with husbandry, medicine and surgery of reptiles—veterinarians, animal keepers, research and educational institutions, herpetologists and sophisticated amateurs. The author's sense of humor, compassion and philosophy, both as a practical and as a practicing veterinarian and as one much concerned with the threat of extinction facing many species of reptiles throughout the world, makes this very well organized volume a pleasure just to read. The information and the illustrations it contains makes it a *must* reading for all those who treat or keep reptiles and who want to keep them healthy and "contented".

The several bibliographies, conveniently separated into appropriate groupings are, indeed, extensive and will be very useful to those seeking more detailed information in original papers.

This volume fills an obvious long-standing need and will become and remain a major work for a long time to come as well as becoming a model for others to follow. It will be most welcome by all who are concerned with reptiles.

Hopefully, it signifies a positive change in attitude toward improving the care and health of reptiles.

Nathan W. Cohen, A.B., M.A., Ph.D.
Director, Curriculum Development in Science
University of California
Berkeley, California
January 1973

Introduction

In TODAY'S sophisticated veterinary clinical practice, the clinician may be called upon to render advice on the care of almost any species of beastie. The veterinarian who actually enjoys treating anything that walks, crawls, flies or swims may soon develop the expertise which will earn him the respect and referrals from colleagues who would rather not include the myriad feathered and scaly amongst their patients.

It can be a source of immense satisfaction to be able to help in an area which has for too long remained unexplored in many communities. We have made our share of errors, but we have learned from each of them. The challenge of an exploratory celiotomy in a tortoise or alligator must be experienced to be appreciated fully.

It was not always possible or desirable to demarcate clearly between animal husbandry and medicine; therefore, some overlapping was unavoidable.

No mention was made of the Tuatara (*Sphenodon punctatum*), a lonely lizard-like reptile which lives on a group of small islands off the main island of New Zealand. This animal is the last survivor of the order *Rhyncocephalia*. Actually, it is not a lizard, but rather a more direct descendant of earlier primitive reptiles from which many of the now-extinct prehistoric forms evolved.

This 1½-foot-long survivor of bygone primeval times is vigorously protected in its native habitat by the New Zealand government. Therefore, the opportunity for the Tuatara to become a captive in a reptile collection fortunately is a remote possibility.

Because of the environmentally- and ecologically-aware society in which we live, perhaps it is appropriate to state that while I prefer to see animals in their native habitat, unrestrained by cages, it is nonetheless obvious that man has always (and probably will always) subject lesser species to various degrees of captivity. While I do not condone such action, I must not fail to render what service I can to help preserve such captive creatures in a state of health and (modified) well being. It was for this reason that this book was written.

Acknowledgments

SINCE this volume is probably the first reptile medicine and surgery text ever written specifically for the practicing veterinary clinician, I have had to draw heavily upon my own experiences.

I would not have had much experience to draw upon had it not been for the unselfish cooperation of practitioner colleagues in the San Francisco Bay area who referred many interesting cases to me. To these fellow professionals I am deeply indebted. The able staff of Steinhart Aquarium, Golden Gate Park, San Francisco—especially Messrs. Glenn Burghardt, Karl Switak, and Robert Dempster—sent me dozens of reptilian patients. Mr. Paul Hoekenga of Marine World/Africa U.S.A. also referred many cases.

Other veterinarians who have greatly contributed to our particular discipline are Dr. Joel Wallach of the Chicago Zoological Park, Brookfield, Illinois, and Dr. Leonard C. Marcus of Boston, Massachusetts.

Dr. Ronald Cauble of the East Bay Vivarium, one of the more enlightened reptile dealer-entrepreneurs, was very kind in referring patients to me, and also made much clinical material from his own stock available to me.

Doctors Jan F. Detrick, Scott H. Schelling, and William D. Loughman deserve special thanks. Jan Detrick helped with many of the electrocardiographic studies, and Scott Schelling was ever ready to assist with dissections and just about anything else. Will Loughman not only allowed me ready access to his photomicrographic laboratory, but gave unselfishly of his time and considerable talents.

Dr. John D. Carney, pathologist at Eden Hospital Laboratories, Castro Valley, California, has shown keen interest in reptilian pathology. I would like to acknowledge his considerable assistance in describing several histopathologic conditions seen in captive reptiles.

The veterinary aide staff of the Berkeley Dog & Cat Hospital was always available and willing to assist me with some of the rather unpleasant chores associated with this type of clinical practice. Their enthusiasm is deeply appreciated.

A special note of gratitude to my publisher, Dr. C. M. Cooper, who made this book ultimately possible. I wanted to include as many color illustrations as practicable, and Dr. Cooper generously accepted this premise.

Mr. Ray E. Ottinger, Jr., who acted as senior editor of this manuscript, brought to his task the genuine enthusiasm and elan which I feel immeasurably improved the final product. The original intent was to employ a concise format which could readily serve as a reference text. Mr. Ottinger certainly contributed to this effort with his expertise.

Lastly, my wife Brucye deserves nothing less than a peerage. Not only has she cheerfully allowed any number of scaly creatures to be housed under the same roof with our family, but she also typed and helped edit this manuscript. Her many suggestions have contributed to the final product and also to the enjoyment of writing it. I am a very fortunate fellow!

The pathology was supported in part by Grant No. Ca. 12490, from the National Cancer Institute, and awarded to the Alameda-Contra Costa County Animal Neoplasm Registry.

Fredric L. Frye, D.V.M.
Kensington, California
September, 1972

HUSBANDRY

A. Housing

Housing must allow for natural habitation proclivities for each species—aquatic, subterranean, and arboreal—with suitable substrates provided, *ie.*, sand or litter for desert or burrowing reptiles; climbing branches for tree dwellers, etc.

The choice of suitable material for cage litter is wide. Each substrate has its advantages and disadvantages. Ready availability, cost, appearance, absorptive qualities, tendency to become ingested with the captive reptile's food or to produce impactions must all be considered. Ground corn cob, sphagnum or peat moss, wood chips or sawdust, sand, various sizes of gravel, newspaper and butcher's paper all have been used. Requirements for each specimen should be considered individually.

Species that dwell on the forest floor should be provided with as natural a habitat as possible; pieces of bark, leaf litter, etc. should be present as cage enrichment.

Many burrowing species may not be visible as often as might be desired if they are provided with an adequate substrate. A trade-off between optimal husbandry practice and public display sometimes must be made.

For those mostly-aquatic species—exemplified by turtles, water monitors, water snakes, etc. — an attractive yet health-promoting environment can be provided by suitable aquarium tanks partially filled with clean water. Cage-enriching items such as branches, rocks, floats, etc. should be available to allow the specimens the opportunity to "haul out" from time to time. Living edible plants may also be included if desired.

In the case of small specimens, waste disposal can be handled adequately with aquarium filtration systems. In larger aquatic environmental displays, more elaborate water filters must be employed. It is absolutely essential that fecal and food wastes not be allowed to accumulate. If natural food items are fed, less waste will result since the prey will usually remain alive until consumed.

B. Water and Humidity

Many rain-forest reptiles will not drink from water containers and must lap droplets from vegetation. Water-mist guns are valuable for providing aerosols. Foliage in the cage should be sprayed twice daily.

Other reptiles will drink readily from suitable water containers. These containers should be large enough to accommodate the entire body of the specimen without causing the water to spill over and dampen the cage litter.

Generally, a 35% to 60% relative humidity is adequate for most species. The higher humidity is essential for some forest dwellers and tropical or semiaquatic species. Desert-dwelling species require much less humidity, but frequently will immerse themselves in deep water containers. Gila monsters with algae-covered backs are a common sight in collections of reptiles. Immersion also aids in skin shedding, especially in snakes.

Too high a humidity, or frank dampness, predisposes many captive reptiles to "blister disease," manifested early as fluid-filled vesicles which soon become secondarily infected and filled with caseated pus (*Figures 1a-1d*).

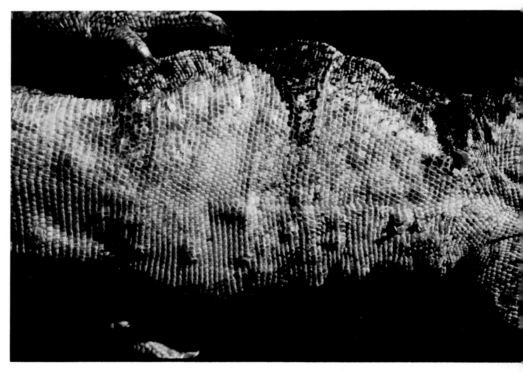

Figure 1a—Blister disease in a lizard. Note the multiple pustules on the ventral side.

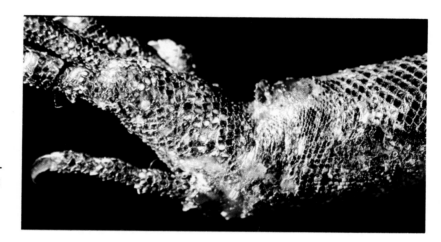

Figure 1b—A close-up photograph of the rear foot from the same lizard.

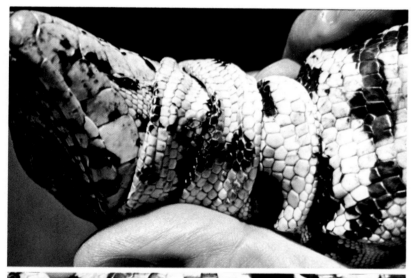

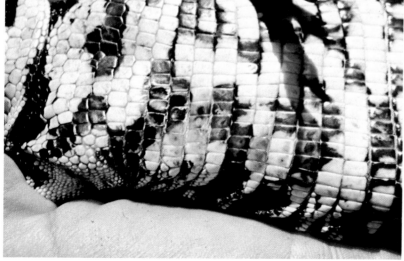

Figures 1c & 1d—Cutaneous infection in a tegu lizard resulting from a cage environment which was too moist and contaminated with feces.

C. Temperature

Dr. Joel Wallach has published temperature requirements for reptiles. The following data are abstracted from his excellent paper (*JAVMA 159:*1632-1643; 1969).

	Range of Active Reptiles	Preferred Optimum	Critical High
American alligator	26.0- 37.0°C (78.0- 98.0° F)	32.0- 35.0°C (89.6- 95.0° F)	38.0- 39.0° C (100.4-102.2° F)
Garter snake	16.0- 34.6°C (60.8- 94.0° F)	22.0- 31.0°C (71.6- 87.8° F)	40.5° C (104.9° F)
Green iguana	26.7- 42.4°C (79.7-108.5° F)	29.5- 39.5°C (85.1-103.1° F)	46.1° C (114.8° F)
Painted turtle	8.0- 30.2°C (46.4- 86.0° F)	23.0- 27.8°C (73.5- 84.0° F)	39.0- 41.0° C (102.2-105.8° F)
Desert tortoise	19.0- 37.8°C (66.2-100.4° F)	26.7- 29.4°C (80.6- 85.1° F)	39.5- 43.0° C (103.1-109.0° F)

If additional warmth is desired, a heat lamp or incandescent light bulb, suitably shielded, may be placed in or near the cage.

A useful alternative to the heat lamp is the use of heating coils or thermal pads under the cage or litter. The resultant heat is more evenly distributed and is far safer once the heat source has been calibrated and adjusted. In small terraria, heating pads work well when put beneath cages that have been elevated on corner blocks or spacers to allow for air circulation. (*See drawing on facing page.*)

The automatic thermostat selector of the heating pad should be started at the lowest setting to avoid inadvertent overheating of the specimen. If necessary, higher settings may be selected gradually, allowing sufficient time for temperature equilibration to occur.

D. Photoperiod

The photoperiod varies greatly with the species. However, a practical solution has been to use a 14-hour light cycle:10-hour dark cycle. Ideally, this interval should be gradually increased and decreased according to the prevailing seasonal changes of natural light and dark. This may be done automatically with home-constructed timing devices. If natural sunlight is provided, some source of shade must be made available. Reptiles do not possess an efficient thermoregulatory mechanism; therefore, they cannot tolerate severe extremes of temperature.

Lizards employ a panting respiration when they are slightly overheated, and will stand with their bodies away from hot surfaces. They will also incline their bodies toward or away from the sun to absorb or reflect radiant solar energy more efficiently. Some species are capable of expanding and contracting melanophore-rich areas of their skin so as to absorb or reflect radiant energy. The pineal gland may act as an endocrine organ in this process.

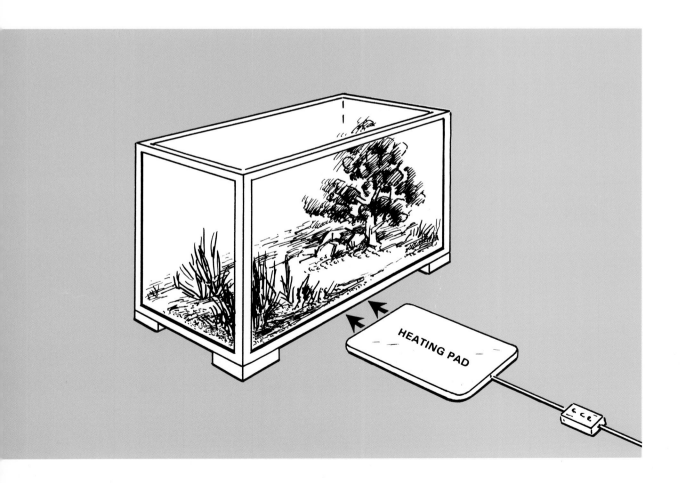

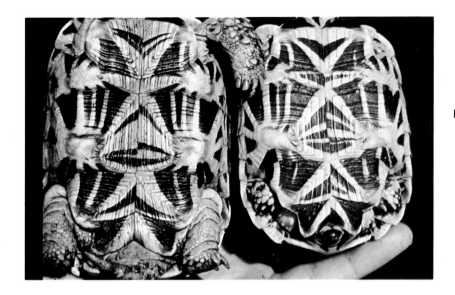

Figure 2a—A male (left) and female (right) star tortoise as viewed from the underside. Note the concave plastron and longer tail of the male. The surface of the plastron in the female is flat.

Figure 2b—A male redfooted tortoise. Note the extreme concavity of the plastron.

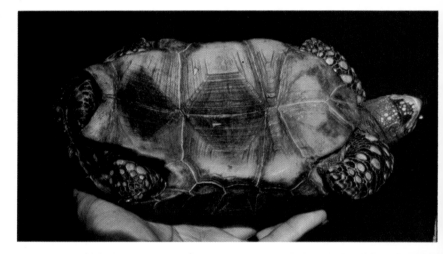

Figure 2c—A female redfooted tortoise.

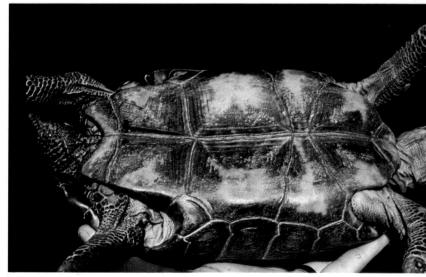

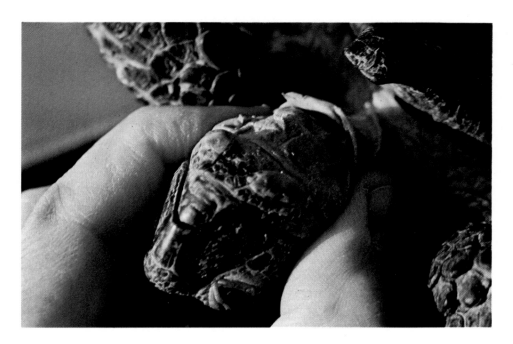

Figure 3—The sexual tubercles are well developed in many tortoises.

E. Reproduction

One of the major goals of husbanding any captive wild species should be reproduction.

1. Sex Identification and Sexual Dimorphism

With few exceptions, observable differences between the sexes are minimal in reptiles. Generally speaking, most chelonian females have a plastron which, when viewed from the side, appears to be almost flat, whereas in males the plastron tends to be rather concave or "dished" (*Figures 2a-2c*). Also, the tail of a female turtle generally is longer and more slender than that of a male of the same size and species. Male tortoises of some species possess well-developed sexual tubercles on either side of the ventral surface of the mandibles (*Figure 3*). These tubercles are thought to be modified scent and tactile organs.

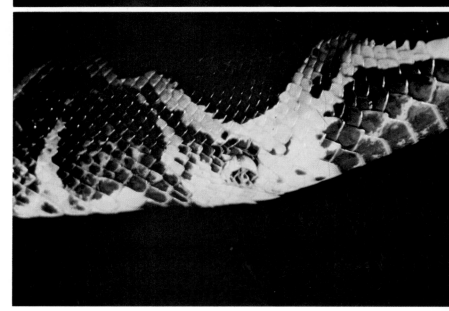

Figure 4a—Area of the cloacal vent in a female boa constrictor.

Figure 4b—Area of the cloacal vent in a male boa constrictor. Note the curved spur which is more prominent in the male.

Boas and pythons usually can be easily sexed by observing the development of the spurs on either side of the cloacal vent (*Figures 4a & 4b, 5a & 5b*). These appendages are remnants of pelvic limbs. The males of these snakes possess larger, more prominent spurs than do females of equal size.

Some iguanid lizards can be sexed by the operculum on either side of the head just caudo-ventral to the tympanum. Males have correspondingly larger shields than females of like size. The dorsal spines also tend to be more heavily developed in the males.

Generally, the coloring of male lizards of the brightly-colored species will be more vivid than that of their female partners.

Some crocodilian species can be sexed by comparing the size of two large swellings just caudal to the eyes. Those in the males will be found to be the larger.

Male snakes and lizards possess paired copulatory organs called *hemipenes*.

Male turtles, tortoises and crocodilia are equipped with one intromittent organ. The male turtle will frequently extend its penis during voiding. The penis of the turtle is, characteristically, a heavily-pigmented, spade-shaped fleshy mass (*Figure 6*).

2. *Intersexuality*

Most reptiles possess a relatively low chromosome number with a diploid number between the limits of 36 and 46. Sex linkage

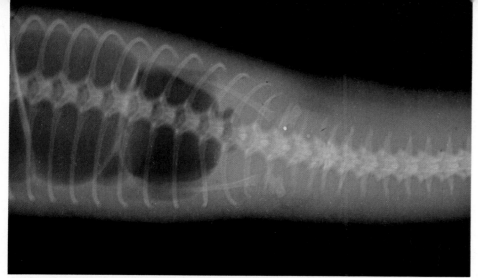

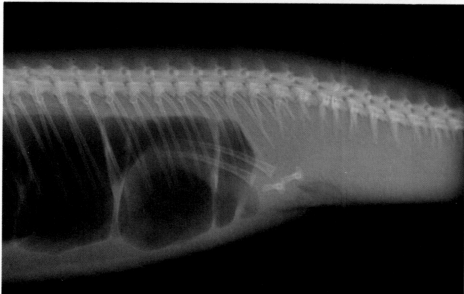

Figures 5a & 5b—Dorsoventral and lateral radiographs of the male boa constrictor shown in Figure 4b. Note the vestigial remnants of a pelvis.

Figure 6—Partially extended penis of the turtle.

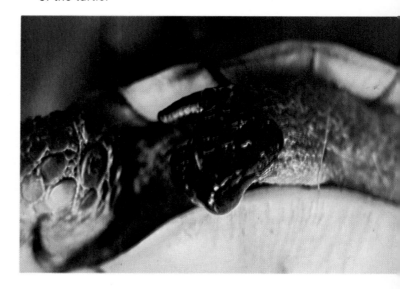

is unknown and there is therefore no genetic evidence of sex chromosomes. It has been shown on endocrinologic grounds that the female might be the heterogametic sex in reptiles; as in birds, however, sex dimorphism in sex chromatin has not as yet been seen in reptiles.

Polyspermy is a normal feature of fertilization in reptiles. Female snakes and lizards store sperm. Fertilization may occur months after the last contact with a fertile and sexually active male of the species.

Parthenogenesis has been reported in reptiles. In considering how an all-female race can reproduce, gynogenesis must be excluded, since bisexually reproducing subspecies, though known, have had no access to all-female subspecies. Immature and mature females of the *Armeniaca* subspecies, isolated from male lizards of any kind, produce all-female progeny. Reptiles and birds are the only amniotes in which adult parthenogenesis has been reported to occur. It should be noted that parthenogenesis in reptiles (lizards) seems to produce only females, whereas in birds (turkeys) the offspring are all males. From this, one would conclude that either the parthenogenesis arises by different cytologic mechanisms in the two groups or that the heterogametic sex is, after all, not the same in reptiles and birds (Beatty, 1964).

Some reptiles are easily encouraged to reproduce in captivity. Others are rarely, if ever, successfully bred. Factors such as territoriality, population density, temperature, humidity, nutrition, photoperiodicity, nesting substrate, etc. all enter into the problem. Each individual species should be considered separately, and its natural habitat and diet should be approximated if practicable. There are a few generalizations which can be made.

Reptiles may be either viviparous (or ovoviviparous) or oviparous. Most reptilian eggs, excepting those of chelonians (turtle, tortoise, terrapin), are pliant and leathery when deposited. A hatching medium may be dampened sand or sphagnum moss contained in earthenware crocks or glass jars. Incubation temperatures are less critical than for birds. Generally speaking, an ambient temperature of 74° F. to 82° F. is sufficient to successfully hatch out fertile reptilian eggs. The eggs should *not* be turned or rotated during incubation.

The eggs of serpentine, saurian and crocodilian species enlarge markedly during fertile incubation. They also become somewhat discolored.

The newly-born or hatched reptile should have a diet which is tailored to its nutritional requirements and size. Insects, baby mice, small lizards, snakes, birds or eggs may be required for those species which must eat whole live food. This is particularly the case with snakes.

Often it is possible to train these neonate reptiles to eat non-living food if the scent of an appropriate prey is rubbed on the proffered food item. If fish or frog slime is rubbed on a young mouse before it is offered as food, the mouse may be made to appear as a fish or frog to snakes that eat only fish or anurans.

The snake selects its food mostly by detection of scent rather than by sight. The initial attack may follow sighting of the prey, but subsequent olfaction and organoleptic sensing is essential. The tongue carries scent particles to the well-developed Jacobson's organ where it is detected, then to the central nervous system where integrated purposeful response is initiated through motor pathways.

F. Cannibalism

Some degree of cannibalism in almost all the reptiles is essentially normal feeding behavior in the strict definitive sense. Many snakes eat only other snakes. When a species consumes members of its *own* species, it must be considered an abnormal trait.

Overcrowded conditions, with the resultant stress of high population density, probably is the major inciting cause of cannibalism. Reducing the population and providing hiding places usually will eliminate this problem. Prey species must not be housed with their predators.

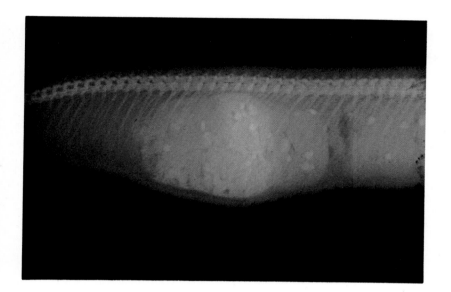

Figure 7—Obstipation in a python. Multiple tricolithous fecal masses can be seen on the radiograph.

G. Vomiting

A frequently-encountered management problem in maintaining captive reptiles, particularly snakes, is vomiting. The two most common causes have been found to be:

1) handling of the specimen after it has eaten,
2) improper ambient temperatures.

Since, in mammal-eating species, the process of digestion may be rather prolonged due to the considerable bulk of the prey, any disturbance of the snake after it has eaten may result in almost immediate vomiting of the last meal. Digestion *per se* is a chemical process greatly dependent upon enzymatic action as well as specific acid- and buffer-containing secretions. These digestive enzymes possess individual activity curves which are highly temperature-dependent. With a significant drop in ambient temperature, there is a corresponding diminution of digestive activity. Frequently, the result is putrefaction rather than digestion of the ingested prey. When this occurs, the partially-digested gastric contents are cast up.

Treatment consists of restricted postprandial handling and the maintenance of optimum ambient temperatures.

Other less common causes for vomiting are gastrointestinal parasitism, intra- and extramural obstruction, infection, neoplasia, etc.

If any of these conditions are found to be the cause, remedial action should eliminate the vomiting. Routine microscopic fecal and sputum examinations, specific treatment, radiographic surveys, and/or surgery may help to diagnose and resolve this problem.

H. Obstipation/Constipation

A captive reptile occasionally will be presented with a complaint from the owner or animal-keeper that the animal is constipated. Much of this problem stems from improper diet and insufficient exercise. Snakes fed a diet of numerous heavily-furred rodents or thickly-feathered birds may produce rather large tricholith-like fecal masses. These masses can be palpated easily and will show clearly on radiographs (*Figure 7*).

Treatment consists of the oral administration of stool-softening agents, especially dioctyl sodium sulfosuccinate (D.S.S. Capsules — Hall Drug Co.). In the case of snakes with fur-laden fecal masses, cloacal instillation of either a fluid containing D.S.S. or water-soluble lubricating jelly usually will help soften the stool bolus and facilitate its passage. Gentle palpation or milking action by the operator usually is an aid in removing these masses. In difficult cases, a long forceps may be required to accomplish the removal.

I. Nutrition

1. Inanition

Many of the reptilian patients seen in practice are presented in a state of virtual starvation-dehydration cachexia (*Figures 8a-8f*). As stores of body fat and muscle are catabolized, the eyes sink, the skin shrivels and the bones become prominent. At best, these patients are extremely labile. Many have not eaten voluntarily in months. Their resistance to stress is almost *nil*. Gentle handling and a quiet environment are almost as essential as nutritonal replacement.

The quickest, most efficient method for immediate restoration of positive lipid, protein and vitamin balance is by tube-feeding with a nutritional-replacement product that has a high-caloric, low-bulk formula designed for convalescent animals (Pet Kalorie®—Haver-Lockhart; Nutrical®—EVSCO). These prod-

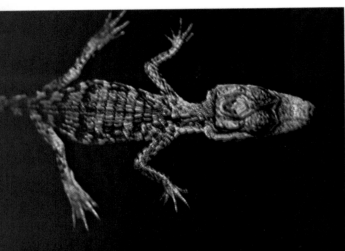

Figure 8a—Inanition-starvation in a caiman.

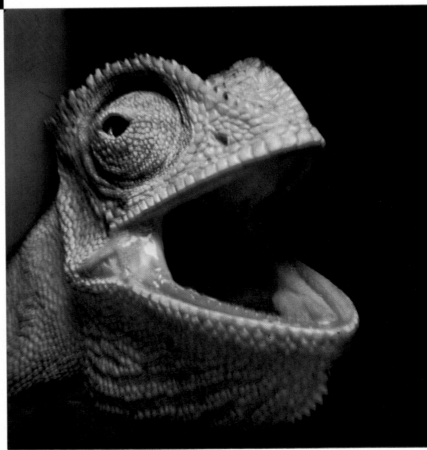

Figure 8b—Inanition-starvation in a chameleon. Note the sunken appearance of the eye and the wrinkling of the skin.

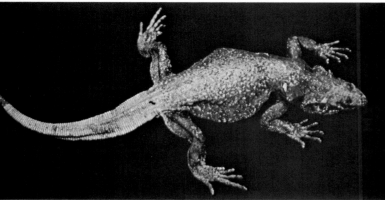

Figure 8c—Inanition-starvation in a chuckwalla.

Figure 8d—Inanition-starvation in a boa constrictor. Note the loss of muscle mass.

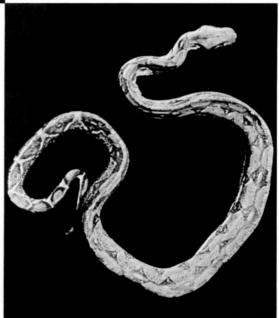

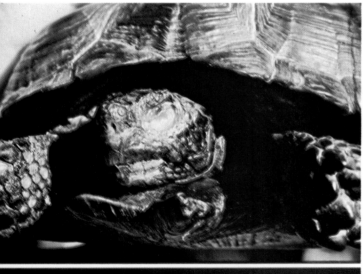

Figure 8e—Inanition-starvation in a tortoise.

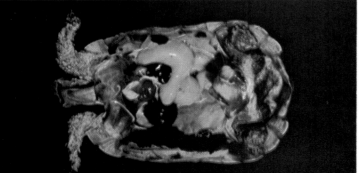

Figure 8f—Extreme degree of tissue loss in a tortoise cadaver. Note the almost total absence of visceral fat. Dehydration is also seen in most of these patients.

Figures 9a & 9b
Dorsoventral and lateral views of a *Pseudemys* turtle with nutritional osteoporosis. Note the misshapen shell. The rear legs are immobile because of pathologic fractures resulting from attempted weight-bearing.

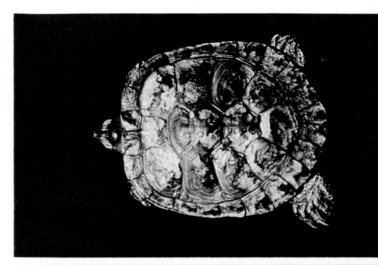

Figure 10a
Dorsoventral radiograph of the turtle seen in Figure 9a. Note the poor ossification of skeletal elements and the pathologic fractures of the long bones.

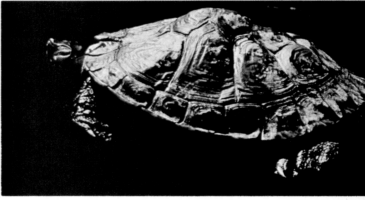

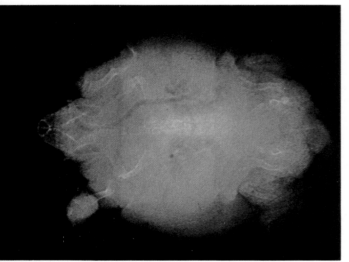

Figure 10b
Dorsoventral radiograph of a normal *Pseudemys*. Compare with Figure 10a.

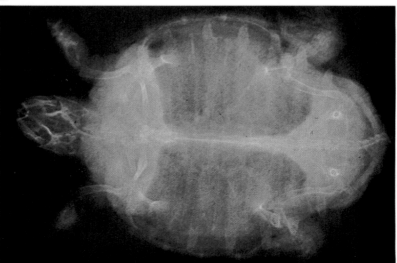

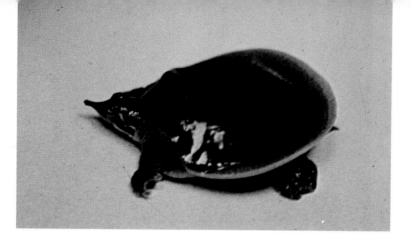

Figure 11
Marked shell curvature in a young *Trionyx* solf-shelled turtle fed a calcium-deficient diet.

ucts may be mixed with pureed infant-food meat diets. A urethral catheter of appropriate size, or an infant-feeding tube, works well for intubation. Both will fit on a syringe with a Luer tip.

If the patient is not eating voluntarily, attempts to hand-feed a natural diet (young mice, rats, baby chicks, etc.) should be made as soon as possible. Food for snakes should be lubricated with beaten egg. Lizards and the chelonia may also be hand-fed appropriate materials. The mouth is opened and small amounts of food are introduced and advanced down the esophagus with a smooth-tipped flexible probe. Plastic artificial insemination pipettes are ideal for this purpose. Gentleness is essential! The single occipital condyle can be easily disarticulated from the atlas. A snake's body should be well supported during handling.

2. Calcium:Phosphorus Imbalance

The calcium:phosphorus ratio is of major clinical significance. The proper balance lies between 1 to 1.5:1.0. The most common imbalance in turtles and iguanas results from a diet containing either too much lean meat or lettuce. In these cases the ratio may be as unbalanced as 1:40 plus. The condition may be further aggravated by a vitamin D deficiency, since most captive reptiles do not receive sufficient ultraviolet radiation.

Bony tissues become so depleted that skeletal deformities result. Frequently, the appendicular skeleton of turtles suffers pathologic fractures through weight-bearing. Later, softening of the shell becomes marked. If the turtle survives, the shell tends to curl, the internal organs become crowded, and debility is further exaggerated (*Figures 9a & 9b, 10a & 10b, 11, 12a & 12b*).

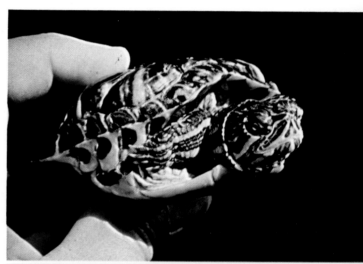

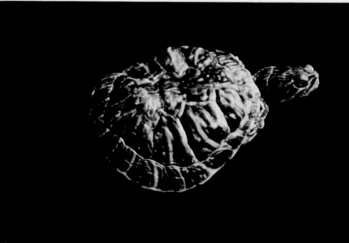

Figures 12a & 12b—Severe shell deformity in a *Pseudemys* after several years of a calcium-deficient diet followed by an adequate calcium-phosphorus intake. Note the stunted size.

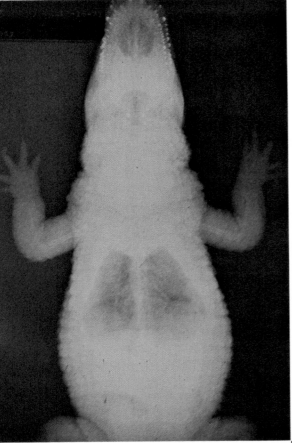

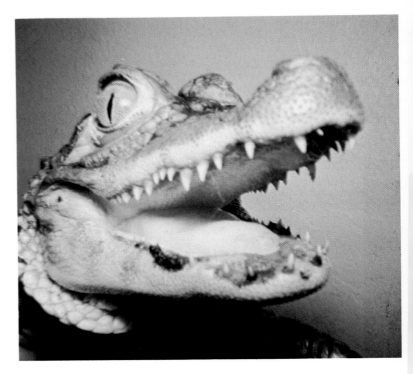

Figure 13—Anterolateral view of a caiman affected with secondary nutritional osteoporosis. Note the foreshortened mandible. This deformity is seen early in the disease and may become extreme in untreated animals.

Figure 14a—Radiograph of nutritional osteoporosis in a young caiman fed a diet of raw meat.

Figure 14b—Pretreatment and post-treatment radiographs of the same caiman. The two radiographs were taken three and one-half months apart. Note the increase in size and degree of ossification that have occurred.

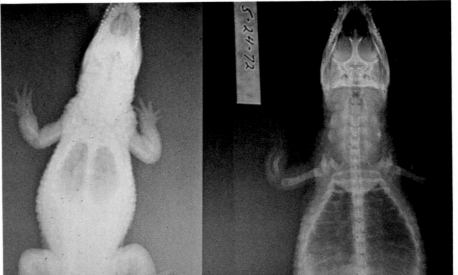

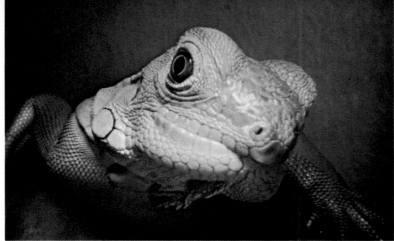

Figures 15a & 15b—Anterior and lateral views of a young iguana suffering from fibrous osteodystrophy. Note the misshapen mandible.

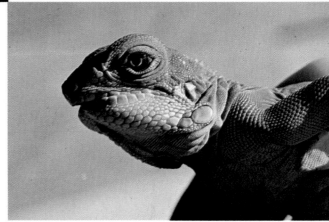

Figures 15c & 15d—Fibrous osteodystrophy in two iguanas. Note the swollen appearance of the limbs, particularly the hindlimbs.

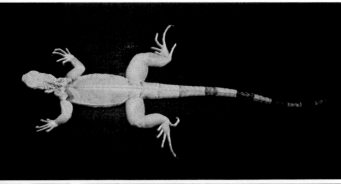

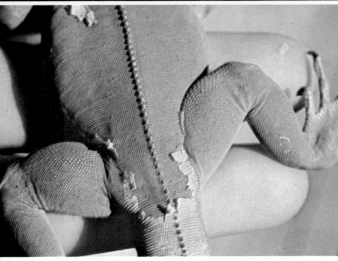

Calcium:phosphorus imbalance is also encountered in captive caimans fed a meat diet without additional calcium (*Figures 13, 14a & 14b*).

Fibrous osteodystrophy is a commonly-presented disorder in iguanas. The outstanding findings consist of markedly firm, swollen limbs and tail. Superficially, the gross appearance is that of a well-fed, chubby lizard (*Figures 15a-15d, 16a & 16b, 17, 18a & 18b, 19*). The owner usually mentions that the iguana's diet has consisted of mainly lettuce and fruit.

Therapy consists of:

1) appropriate injections of calcium gluconate two or three times weekly;
2) oral vitamin D and calcium supplementation;
3) a change of diet to one which is more natural for the particular species.

Figure 16a—Radiograph of the normal hindlimbs and tail in an iguana.

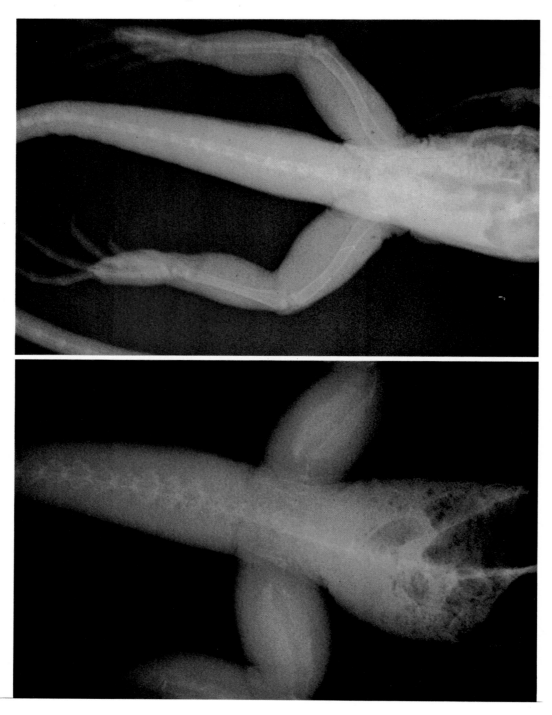

Figure 16b—Radiograph of an iguana with fibrous osteodystrophy. Note the irregular "motheaten" appearance of the long bones and coccygeal elements. The diameter of the marrow cavities in the femurs is essentially normal.

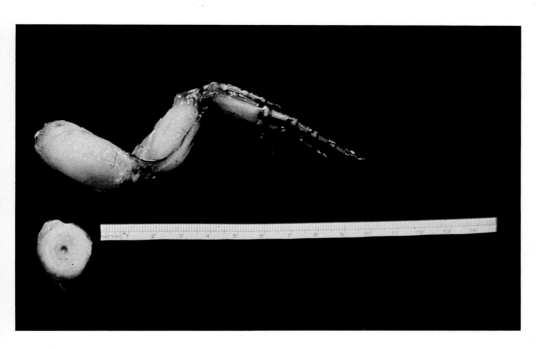

Figure 17
Postmortem specimens from the osteodystrophic iguana shown in Figure 15d.

Figures 18a & 18b—Osteologic preparations of bones seen in Figure 17. Note the spongy appearance of the bony tissue.

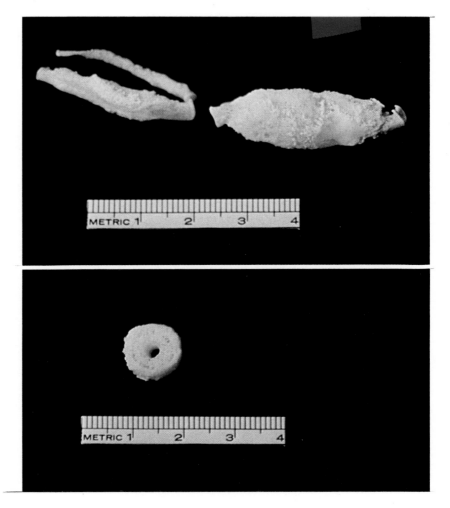

For aquatic turtles, the corrective diet should include: earthworms; whole (preferably live) fish such as mosquito fish, sticklebacks or goldfish; green leafy vegetation such as watercress, romaine lettuce, swiss chard, etc. A proper diet for iguanas should include: young mice, crickets, mealworms, dandelion flowers, rose petals, carnations, and thawed frozen mixed vegetables.

Frozen fish or fish not recently killed may contain significant levels of the enzyme thiaminase. Therefore, if thiamine deficiency is to be avoided, exogenous thiamine should be provided. There is also a threat of induced steatitis in captive reptiles—particularly in caimans, alligators and crocodiles—if a fish diet is fed exclusively. Small mice or chicks are an excellent dietary supplement for these species.

These crocodilia are also subject to fasting

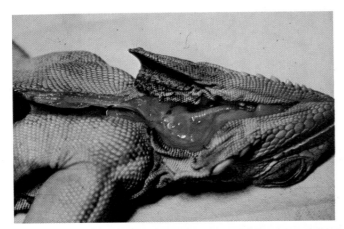

Figure 19—Postmortem specimen of an iguana. Note the hyperplastic parathyroid glandular tissue.

Figure 20—Visceral and skeletal gout in an iguana. Note the radiopaque lesions in the liver and gut. There is a small accumulation of uric acid crystals in the left axilla.

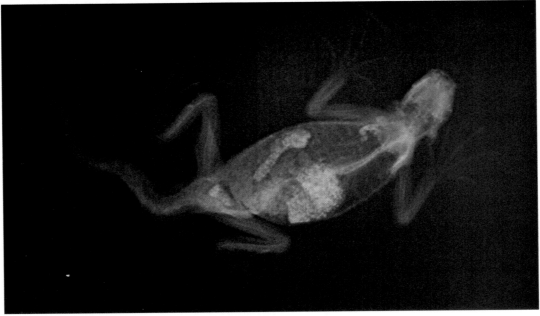

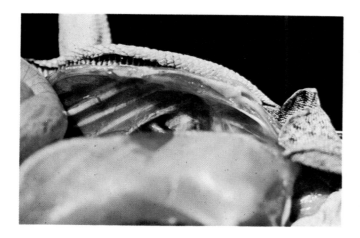

Figure 21—Postmortem specimen from the iguana shown in Figure 20. Note the gouty tophi between the ribs.

Figures 22a & 22b—Visceral gout in a caiman. Uric acid crystalline material in the pericardium and liver is seen as small light lesions.

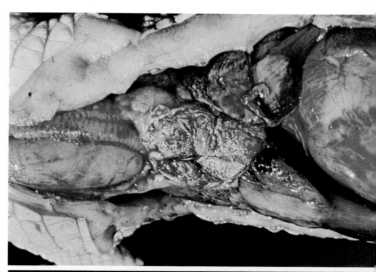

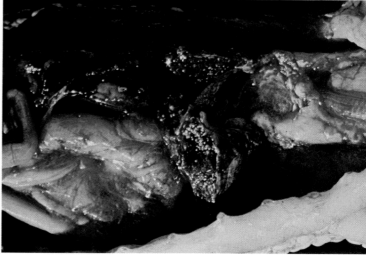

and stress-induced hypoglycemia. Typical signs are tremors, slow or absent righting reflex, and torpor. One consistent finding has been mydriasis. Treatment is the administration of oral glucose at the rate of 3 Gm./kg. bodyweight, and the removal of the stressful conditions.

Some natural source of sunlight radiation is desirable. However, artificial ultraviolet fluorescent lamps (Grolux®—Sylvania; Vita-Lite® —Durotest Corp., North Bergen, N.J.) will produce sufficient ultraviolet radiation of the appropriate wave length to produce irradiated ergosterol.

3. Visceral Gout and "Renal Constipation"

Visceral gout and "renal constipation" are frequently found in captive iguanas, tegus, tortoises and crocodilia. The cause is usually a diet which is too high in protein *per se* or contains an excess of organ meat. Water deprivation, with resultant incomplete clearance of uric acid, also has been suggested as the principal cause of renal constipation.

Lesions of this disease may be seen on routine radiographs and postmortem examinations. Deposits of uric acid have been observed in the pericardium, epicardium, myocardium, liver, kidneys and extravisceral sites (*Figures 20, 21, 22a & 22b*). When examined under polarized light microscopy, the uric acid crystals appear as birefringent foci. Multinucleated giant cells which form rosettes are a typical feature of histologic sections (*Figures 23a & 23b, 24a-24d*).

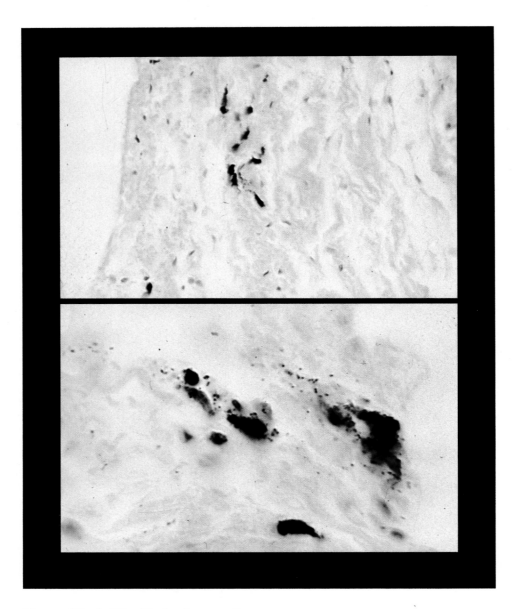

Figures 23a & 23b—Photomicrographs
of a histologic section of a myocar-
dial lesion. Note the dark accumu-
lations of uric acid crystals (H & E
x 100 and 430, respectively).

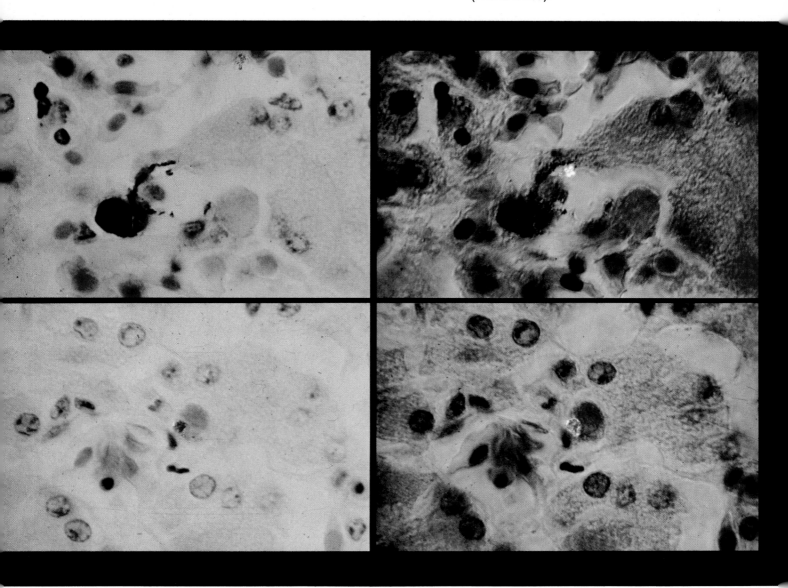

Prevention of uric acid accumulation is afforded by an adequate, balanced (natural) diet and a constantly available source of fresh water. Most desert or gopher tortoises will thrive on a diet of fresh assorted vegetables, fruit, flower petals (rose, carnation, pink or nasturtium), dandelion tops and leaves, small amounts of prepared dog food, bread, etc. Fresh water should be provided *ad libitum*.

Iguanas should be fed assorted fresh fruits and vegetables, flowers, some dog food, and young mice. Monitors and tegus, depending on their size, will do well with a diet consisting of beaten whole egg, chopped lean meat, multivitamin-mineral supplement, mice, rats, and insects such as crickets.

Captive crocodiles should be fed a variety of animal parts and, if possible, an occasional whole mouse, rat or chicken.

4. Hypo- or Avitaminosis A

And the wild asses did stand in the high places, they snuffed up the wind like dragons; their eyes did fail, because there was no grass.
—Chapter 14, Verse 6, of *The Book of Jeremiah.*

This was probably the first published clinical description of hypovitaminosis A.

This syndrome is frequently seen in aquatic turtles, especially during the first year or two of life. The majority of vitamin A storage is hepatic and originates from the embryonic yolk. Unless sources of exogenous carotene or vitamin A are ingested to replace that which is expended in day-to-day metabolism, a state of deficiency eventually results in signs of illness.

Commercial turtle foods are woefully lacking in usable vitamin A. Lettuce has little carotene. Therefore, the usual captive diet of the newly-acquired hatchling (dried ant or termite eggs, lettuce and raw meat) soon depletes any stored hepatic vitamin A. Epithelial tissues rapidly lose their integrity and the ability to resist infection from the many pathogens in the immediate environment. The result is ophthalmic, conjunctival and respiratory infection.

Frequently, the earliest signs of impending hypovitaminosis A crisis are puffy, swollen eyelids, and such respiratory signs as open-mouth breathing, wheezing, nasal discharge, etc. (*Figure 25*).

Therapy consists of either oral or injectable forms of vitamin A. Aquasol-A® (U.S. Vitamin and Pharmaceutical), a water-miscible injectable form, is well tolerated by even the smallest chelonian. Routine, judicious use of ABDEC® Drops (Parke-Davis) is probably justified. Protection against secondary infection should be given by the use of appropriate antibiotics and ophthalmic ointments.

5. Hypo- or Avitaminosis K

This condition reportedly occurs in alligators, caimans, crocodiles and gavials. The first sign of the deficiency I have noted is rather severe gingival bleeding *without* petechiation. As deciduous teeth are shed, there is excessive alveolar bleeding which may continue for days. Injectable vitamin K usually will stop this bleeding quickly.

The diet of the captive crocodilian should be supplemented routinely with oral synthetic vitamin K. This inexpensive preventive measure has completely eliminated the problem.

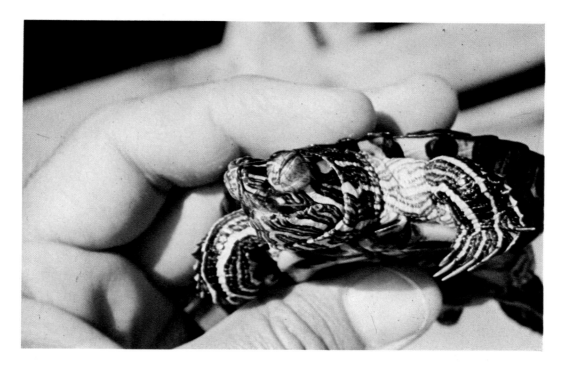

Figure 25—A turtle showing severe blepharitis and conjunctivitis. Typically, these conditions are early signs of hypo- or avitaminosis A. These tissues frequently are secondarily infected.

6. *Hypovitaminosis C*

This vitamin deficiency has recently been reported to occur in snakes and lizards. We have found that snakes, lizards and chelonians with infectious stomatitis respond more quickly when ascorbic acid is added empirically to their antibiotic medication. The dosage used has been a minimum of 25 mg. for small patients, and several grams daily for very large reptiles. Patients have tolerated the treatment well without overt unfavorable reactions.

7. *Steatitis*

Steatitis was mentioned earlier with regard to crocodilia fed oil-laden species of fish. The condition has also been reported to occur in snakes fed obese laboratory rats.

Steatitis is characterized by yellow-to-brown pigmented nodular lesions throughout the subcutaneous and thoracico-abdominal cavity (*Figures 26a-26g*). Adhesions between parenchymatous visceral organs are a consistent finding. Lipid infiltration of the liver is also common. Frequently, the abdominal organs are found to be a solid mass of discolored

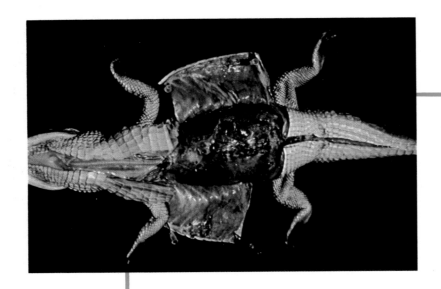

Steatitis
in a Caiman

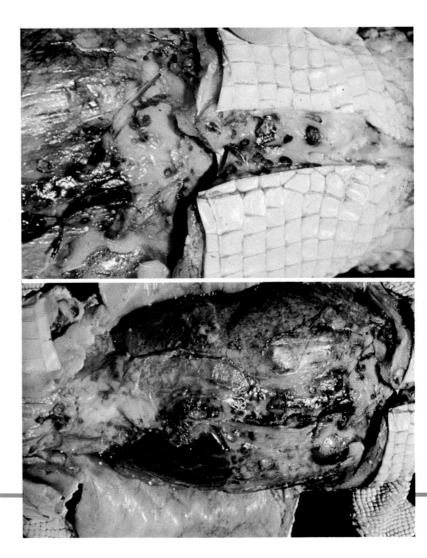

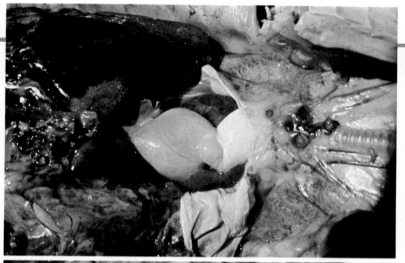

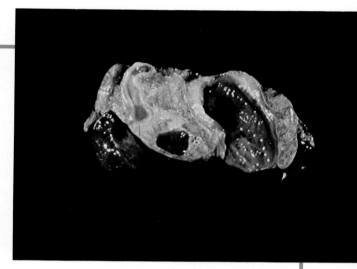

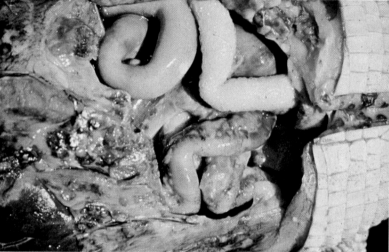

Figures 26a to 26g—Gross pathology in a case of steatitis in a caiman. Note the severe fat necrosis, visceral adhesions, and focal hepatic necrosis. Figure 26g shows a cross-section of the visceral mass at the level of the stomach. The stomach, duodenum, spleen, liver and pancreas can be identified in the section.

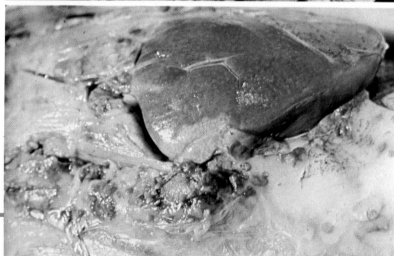

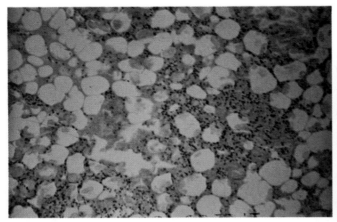

Figure 27a—Photomicrograph of histologic sections of steatitis showing fat. Note the cellular infiltration and ceroid pigment (H & E x 100).

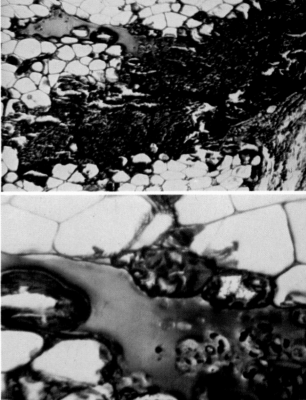

Figures 27b & 27c—Specific staining to illustrate the ceroid pigment characteristic of steatitis. Note the multinucleated giant cells and waxy ceroid (x 100 and 430, respectively).

tissue with little or no separation of identifiable structures. Upon histopathologic examination of sectioned tissues, the typical waxy material, ceroid, is found as solid pearls or engulfed in phagocytes and multinucleated giant cells. Cellular infiltration by inflammatory cells is marked (*Figures 27a-27c*).

The pathogenesis of steatitis is thought to be the excessive consumption of unsaturated or rancid fatty acids over a long period of time. Peroxidation of these fatty acids results in the production of ceroid pigment with subsequent inflammatory response. Adequate levels of vitamin E, because of its antioxidant properties, will prevent, and may reverse, some of the described pathologic changes.

If oil-laden animals are to be used routinely for feed, the supplementary use of exogenous vitamin E should be contemplated.

8. *Sodium Chloride*

The need for additional sodium chloride in the diets of reptiles is essentially confined to marine species maintained in fresh water. These animals possess salt glands which actively secrete excessive sodium chloride ingested with food. Even with non-saline ambient water, the secretion of salt by this mechanism does not cease entirely. A small amount of salt added to the diet will ensure sufficient turnover of sodium chloride. There

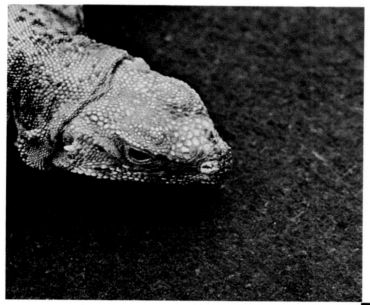

Figure 28—A chuckwalla with a nasal accumulation of sodium chloride crystals.

Figure 29—An iguana showing the typical attitude of posterior limb paresis and tail flaccidity. Empirically, these lizards usually exhibit marked improvement when treated with high levels of multi B-complex vitamins, especially vitamin B_1 (thiamine hydrochloride).

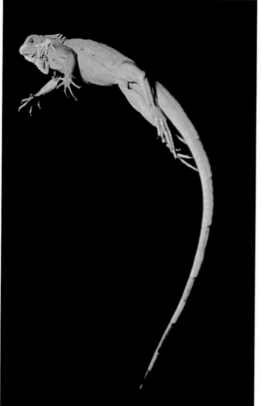

is usually sufficient sodium chloride in the diet of non-marine species. Salt deposits are often seen around the nostrils of desert-dwelling lizards (*Figure 28*).

9. Obesity

Although the majority of nutritional difficulties in captive reptiles are directly associated with malnutrition, insufficiency of total digestible nutrients, or vitamin-mineral deficiencies and/or imbalances, a percentage of these animals will be found to be suffering the effects of too much caloric intake for their particular metabolic requirements. It is not uncommon for a zealous amateur herpetologist to overfeed his pets in an effort to see how fast he can induce them to grow. Without sufficient energy demand on the reptile's metabolism, excess food energy is stored as fat deposits. If this situation continues for enough time, fatty infiltration of parenchymatous visceral organs will occur.

Whereas garter snakes, ringneck snakes, whiptail lizards, etc. should be fed once or twice weekly, a meal every three weeks might

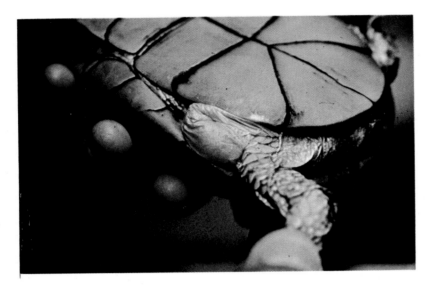

Figure 30—Myxedema-like condition in a box tortoise. Note the swelling just anterior to the hindleg. Supplemental iodine in the diet usually produces a marked reduction of this swelling in a short time.

be more suitable for large pythons and boas. Generally, iguanas and the aquatic chelonians should be fed two or three times weekly. Tortoises apparently tolerate daily self-feeding on vegetation and will thrive if the ambient temperature is sufficiently high to promote activity.

Fasting may be quite prolonged in some reptiles without causing serious effects if the water consumption is adequate to allow for normal renal function. Reptiles have been reported to fast for as long as 36 months without suffering deleterious effects, but such lengthy periods of fasting represent the extreme.

Frozen mixed vegetables are an excellent source of total digestible nutrients, vitamins and minerals for tortoises and iguanas. The vegetables need not be cooked, but they should be thawed thoroughly prior to feeding.

In summary, the prophylactic supplementation of the captive reptile's diet with a balanced preparation yielding calcium, vitamins A, B-complex, C, D, E, and K would seem to be sound practice. In light of the difficulty encountered in attempting to replace many of the exhibit animals presently on the endangered-species list, the practice would also appear to be economically and ecologically beneficial.

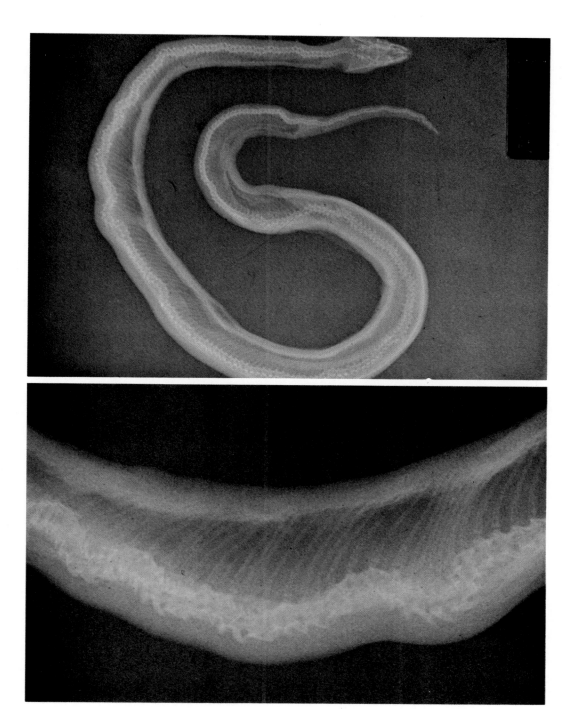

Figures 31a & 31b—Radiographs of skeletal deformities in a young boa constrictor. The suspected cause is a form of muscular dystrophy. Partial recovery was seen after treatment with injectable vitamin E and selenium. Total return to normal was not observed in this boa constrictor.

Bibliography

Appleby, E.C.; Siller, W.G.: Some Cases of Gout in Reptiles. *J. Path. & Bact. 30*:427-430; 1960.

Beatty, R.A.: Chromosome Deviations and Sex in Vertebrates. In *Intersexuality in Vertebrates Including Man,* edited by C.N. Armstrong and A.J. Marshall. Academic Press, London, England, 1964; pp. 101-106.

Benedict, F.G.: *The Physiology of Large Reptiles.* Publication 425, Carnegie Institution, Washington, D.C. 1932.

Bogert, C.M.: Thermoregulation in Reptiles, a Factor in Evolution. *Evolution 3*:195-211; 1949.

Brattstrom, B.H.: Body Temperature in Reptiles. *Am. Midland Nat. 73*:376-422; 1965.

Collins, D.R.: Quantities of Calcium Carbonate Needed to Balance Calcium-Phosphorus Ratios of Various Meats. *J. Zoo Anim. Med. 2*:25; 1971.

Coulson, R.A.; Hernandez, T.: *Biochemistry of the Alligator.* Louisiana State Press, Baton Rouge, La., 1964; pp. 3-6, 76-81.

Cowan, D.F.: Diseases of Captive Reptiles. *JAVMA 153*:848-859; 1968.

Crawford, E.C.: Brain and Body Temperatures in a Panting Lizard. *Science 177*:431-433; 1972.

Dantchakoff, V.: *Arch. Anat. Micr. Morph. Exp. 39*:368-394; 1950.

Darevskii, I.S.: *Doklady Akad. Nauk. S.S.S.R.; 122*: 877-879 of translation Biol. Sci. Sect. Amer. Inst. Biol. Sci., Washington, D.C., 1958.

Dawson, W.L.: Interspecific Variation in Physiological Responses of Lizards to Temperature. In *Lizard Ecology,* edited by W.W. Milstead, University of Missouri Press, Columbia, Mo., 1967; pp. 230-269.

Dunson, W.A.: Reptilian Salt Glands. In *Exocrine Glands,* edited by Botelho, S.Y.; Brooks, F.P.; Shelly, W,H., University of Pennsylvania Press. Philadelphia, Pa., 1969; pp. 89-103.

Evans, H.E.: Keeping Reptiles as Pets. In *Current Veterinary Therapy III,* edited by R.W. Kirk. W.B. Saunders Co., Philadelphia, Pa., 1968; pp. 422-435.

Fox, W.: Special Tubules for Sperm Storage in Female Lizards. *Nature 198*:500-501; 1963.

Frankel, H.M.; Steinberg, G.; Gordon, J.: Effects of Temperature on Blood Gases, Lactate and Pyruvate in Turtles (*Pseudemys scripta elegans*) *in vivo. Comp.*

Biochem. Physiol. 19:279-283; 1966.

Frye, F.L.; Schelling, S.H.; Carney, J.: Steatitis in a Caiman. *Veterinary Med./Small Anim. Clin.* 68:143-145; 1973.

Gandal, C.P.: A Practical Method of Obtaining Blood from Anesthetized Turtles by Means of a Cardiac Puncture. *Zoologica 43:* Nov. 20, 1958.

Gans, C.: *The Biology of the Reptilia, Vol. I and II.* Academic Press, New York, N.Y., 1969.

Gloor, U.; Wiss, O.: Fat-Soluble Vitamins. *Ann. Rev. Biochem.* 33:318-319; 1964.

Heath, J.E.: The Origins of Thermoregulation. In *Evolution and Environment,* edited by Drake, E. Yale University Press, New Haven, Conn., 1968; pp. 259-278.

Hunt, R.H.: Breeding of the Spectacled Caiman (*Camen c. crocodilus*) at Atlanta Zoo. *Internat. Zoo Yearbook* 9:36-37; 1969.

Ippen, R.: Considerations on the Comparative Pathology of Bone Diseases in Reptiles. *Zentralbl. allg. Path.* 108:424-434; 1965.

Kauffeld, C.: The Effect of Altitude, Ultraviolet Light, and Humidity on Captive Reptiles. *Internat. Zoo Yearbook* 9:8-9; 1969.

Laszlo, J.: Observations on Two New Artificial Lights for Reptile Displays. *Internat. Zoo Yearbook* 9:12-13; 1969.

Llewellyn, G.C.: An Automatic and Self-Adjusting Photoperiod Device for Duplicating the External Daylength. *Lab. Anim. Sci.* 22:565-567; 1972.

Maslin, T.P.: All-Female Species of the Lizard Genus, *Cnemidophorus,* Teiidae. *Science* 135:212-213; 1962.

Makino, S.: In *Growth,* edited by Altman, P.L.; Dittmer, D.S. Biological Handbooks. Fed. Soc. Expt'l Biol., Washington, D.C., 1962; pp. 1-7.

McCutcheon, F.H.: The Respiratory Mechanism in Turtles. *Physiol. Zool.* 16:255-269; 1943.

Mertens, R.: *The World of Amphibians and Reptiles.* McGraw-Hill Book Co., New York, N.Y., 1960.

Murphy, J.B.: Notes on Iguanids and Varanids in a Mixed Exhibit at Dallas Zoo. *Internat. Zoo Yearbook* 9:39-41; 1969.

Pawley, R.: Observations on a Prolonged Food Refusal Period of an Adult Fer de Lance (*Bothrops atrox asper.*) *Internat. Zoo Yearbook* 9:58-59; 1969.

Peaker, M.: Some Aspects of the Thermal Requirements of Reptiles in Captivity. *Internat. Zoo Yearbook* 9:3-8; 1969.

Pope, C.H.: *The Reptile World.* Alfred A. Knopf. New York, N.Y., 1960.

Pritchard, P.: *Living Turtles of the World.* T.F.H. Publications, Jersey City, N.J., 1967.

Schmidt, K.P.; Inger, R.F.: *Living Reptiles of the World.* Hanover House, New York, N.Y., 1957.

Schmidt-Nielsen, K.; Fange, R.: Salt Glands in Marine Reptiles. *Nature* 182:783-785; 1958.

Schuchman, S.M.; Taylor, D.O.N.: Arteriosclerosis in an Iguana (*Iguana iguana*). *JAVMA* 157:614-616; 1970.

Shaw, C.E.: Some Remarks on Captive Care of Reptiles. *Trans. of Symp. I. Pet Health and Ecological Studies Fndn.,* Feb. 21, 1971; pp. 3-14.

Wallach, J.D.; Hoessle, C.: Hypervitaminosis D in Green Iguanas. *JAVMA* 149:912-914; 1966.

Wallach, J.D.; Hoessle, C.; Bennett, J.: Hypoglycemic Shock in Captive Alligators. *JAVMA* 151:893-896; 1967.

Wallach, J.D.; Hoessle, C.: Visceral Gout in Captive Reptiles. *JAVMA* 151:897-899; 1967.

Wallach, J.D.; Hoessle, C.: Steatitis in Captive Crocodilians. *JAVMA* 153:845-847; 1968.

Wallach, J.D.; Hoessle, C.: Fibrous Osteodystrophy in Green Iguanas. *JAVMA* 153:863-865; 1968.

Wallach, J.D.: Medical Care of Reptiles, *JAVMA* 155:1017-1034; 1969.

Wallach, J.D.: Nutritional Diseases of Exotic Animals. *JAVMA* 157:583-599; 1970.

Wallach, J.D.: Diseases of Reptiles and Their Clinical Management. In *Current Veterinary Therapy IV,* edited by R.W. Kirk. W.B. Saunders Co., Philadelphia, Pa., 1971; pp. 433-439.

Wallach, J.D.: Environmental and Nutritional Diseases of Captive Reptiles. *JAVMA* 159:1632-1643; 1971.

Webster, T.P.; Hall, W.P.; Williams, E.E.: Fission in the Evolution of a Lizard Karyotype. *Science* 177:611-613; 1972.

Zwart, P.; van der Watering, C.C.: Disturbance of Bone Formation in the Common Iguana (*Iguana iguana, L.*). Pathology and Etiology. *Acta Zoo. et Path. Anat.* 48:336-356; 1969.

MEDICINE

A. Hematology

1. Obtaining Specimens

A nail may be clipped short to obtain a drop or two of blood from small specimens. Cardiac puncture, venipuncture of lateral tail veins and jugular veins may also be employed.

Large volumes of blood may be obtained with ease from the jugular vein of an alligator.

For cardiac puncture in turtles and tortoises, a 1/16-inch hole may be drilled over the large heart, then sealed with epoxy resin after the sample has been obtained (*Figure 32*).

2. Morphology

All reptiles and amphibians possess nucleated red blood cells. There are several types of white blood cells: neutrophil, heterophil, eosinophil, basophil, large and small lymphocytes, and monocyte.

The neutrophil is characterized by a rather large mononuclear leukocyte in which the cytoplasm may contain both slightly fine eosinophilic and azurophilic granules. The nonsegmented nucleus contains a rather coarse chromatin with significant dense clumping interspersed between a fine ground substance. This nonsegmented nucleus can best be described as similar to that seen in mammalian neutrophilic nuclear chroma-

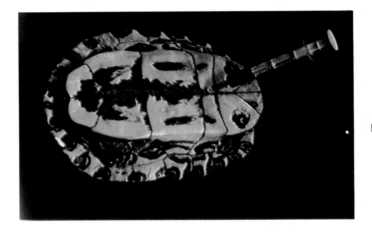

Figure 32—Site of cardiac puncture in the turtle. The area should be prepared as for aseptic surgery by cleansing and the application of an appropriate disinfectant.

tin patterns. The nuclear membrane may be slightly indented or scalloped, but is not truly segmented (*Figure 34a*).

The differentiating feature of the *heterophil* is the presence of elongated rod-shaped granules as opposed to the spherical inclusions seen in the eosinophil. These granules usually stain intermediately between those of the eosinophil and the basophil. The heterophil is more prominent in aquatic chelonians than in other reptiles (*Figure 34c*).

The granulocyte most frequently seen in reptilian blood films is the *eosinophil*. Perhaps this is a reflection of the heavy parasite burden borne by these species. In most cases, the cytoplasm is completely filled with small spherical eosinophilic granules. The small bluish nucleus is usually displaced well to one side of the margin of the cell (*Figures 34d & 34e*).

The *basophil* is also found in large numbers. The deeply-staining basophilic granules usually obscure the more subtle intracellular detail (*Figures 34f & 34g*).

The *lymphocyte* may be either large or small, as in the mammalian species (*Figure 35a*). The cytoplasm is finely granular and basophilic, and it may contain an occasional stained or hyaline inclusion. Juvenile lymphocytes (prolymphocytes) may possess a single well-defined nucleolus.

The reptilian *monocyte* is quite similar to the mammalian variety. It contains a single deeply-indented, centrally-located nucleus with a fine nuclear chromatin pattern. When stained with Wright's stain, the cytoplasm is faintly basophilic-grayish (*Figure 35b*).

The reptilian *thrombocyte* is typically an elliptical cell approximately one-third the size of a mature erythrocyte. The cell has a centrally-located spherical nucleus in which the nuclear chromatin is less dense than that seen in the erythrocyte. The cytoplasm is blue-gray when stained with Giemsa or Wright's stains (*Figures 36a & 36b*). There is much less tendency toward clumping of the thrombocytes in reptilian blood films as compared to those from mammalian species made under the same conditions.

The reptilian *erythrocytic* series is quite similar to that seen in mammals. The major exception is that the mature red cell in reptiles contains a centrally-located, elongated and dense nucleus (*Figure 37*).

Except in severe hematopoietic stress, erythrocytic precursors are limited to polychromatophilic erythrocytes. In the single case (to this date) of myeloproliferative disease in reptiles, stem cells were found as early as proerythroblasts, with a progression from the primordial to the most mature cell types. Obviously, this is an extremely rare finding.

While a true reticulocyte has not been observed in the reptilian erythrocytic series, juvenile erythrocytes are typically seen as slightly larger and somewhat more polychromatophilic when the slide is stained with Giemsa or Wright's stains. When supravitally stained with New Methylene Blue, these cells are frequently found to contain a fine reticulum-like residue within the cytoplasm.

An automatic WBC/RBC counter should not be used. All cells are nucleated, and falsely high readings will result if an automated counter is employed.

Routine staining of blood films with Wright's stain, Giemsa, etc. is satisfactory. I use Gugol's Wright's Stain® (Wampole Laboratories).

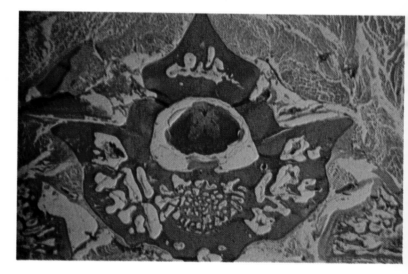

Figure 33—Sites of bone marrow in a snake. This is a whole-mount cross-section of a vertebra from a boa constrictor. Note the marrow-rich areas of the vertebral body (H & E x 5).

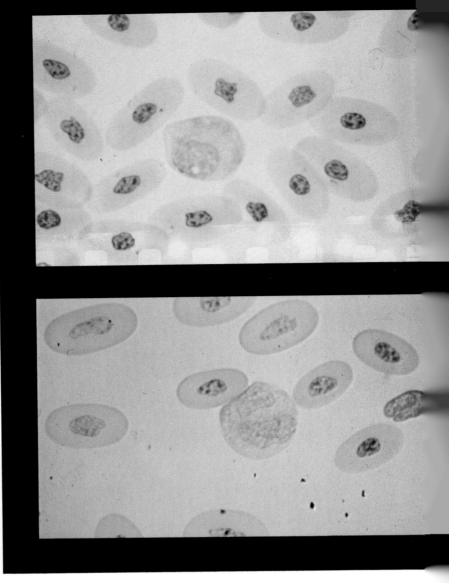

Figure 34a & 34b—Neutrophils from a turtle. (These cells have been shown by specific alkaline phosphatase and peroxidase to be neutrophils.)

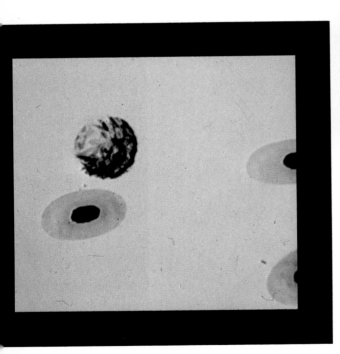

Figure 34c—Heterophil. Note the multiple fusiform intracytoplasmic inclusions.

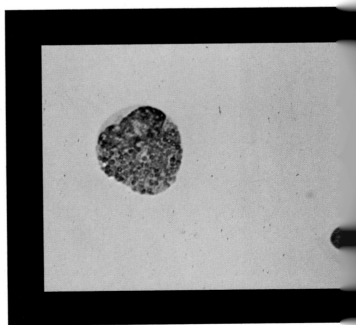

Figure 34d—Eosinophil.

Granulocytic Series (*Figures 34a-34g*)

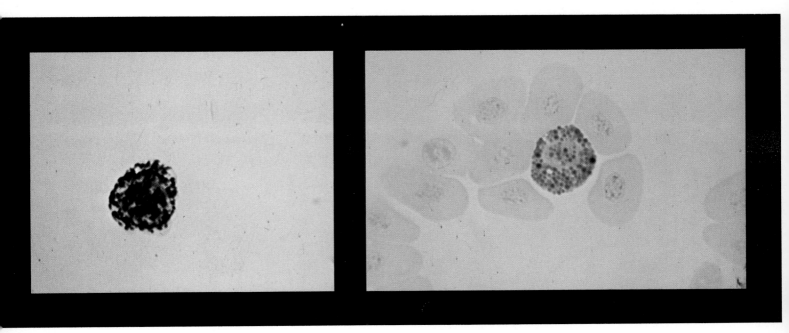

Figure 34f—Basophil from a turtle.

Figure 34g—Basophil from an alligator. The granules usually are somewhat more prominent in crocodilia than in other reptiles.

Figure 34e—Eosinophil as it frequently appears in disease. Note how the granules fail to stain with Wright-type stains. The nucleus is usually eccentrically placed within the eosinophils.

Nongranulocytic Leukocytes (*Figures 35a-35d*)

Figure 35a—Lymphocyte (right-center of field).

Figure 35b—Monocyte.

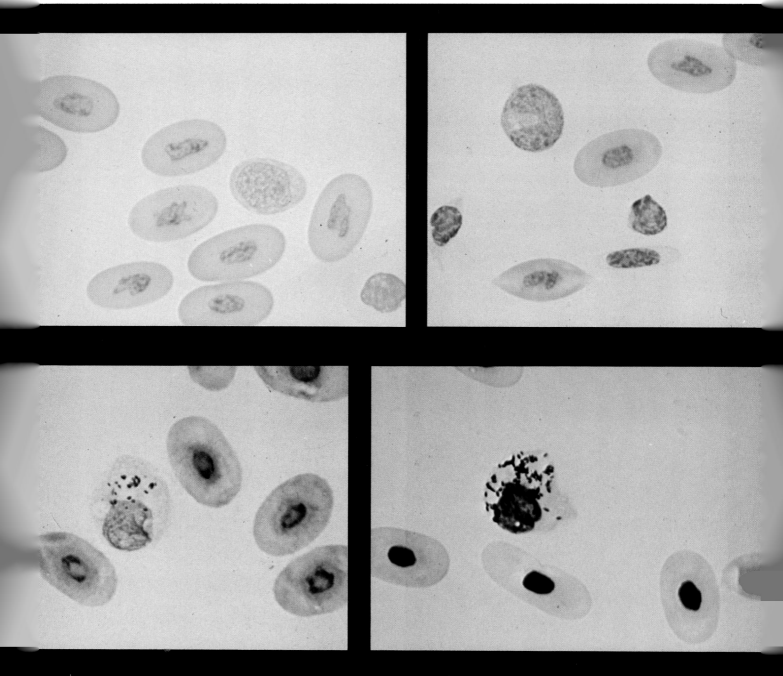

Figures 35c & 35d—Mononuclear cells with engulfed bacteria.

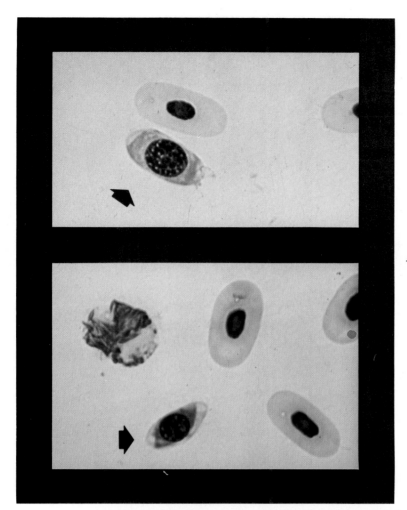

Figures 36a & 36b
Thrombocytes (arrows).

Figure 37
Erythrocytes.

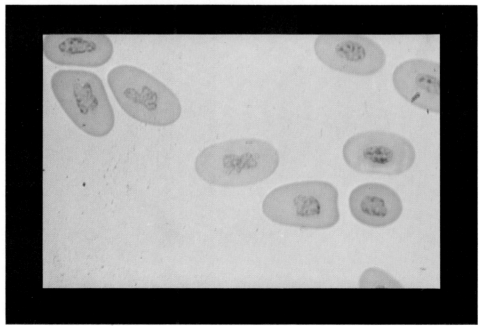

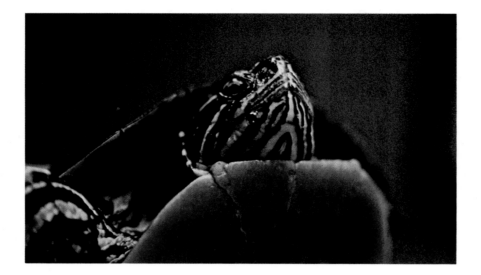

Figure 38a
Respiratory infection in a turtle. Note the bubble at the corner of the mouth and the nasal exudate.

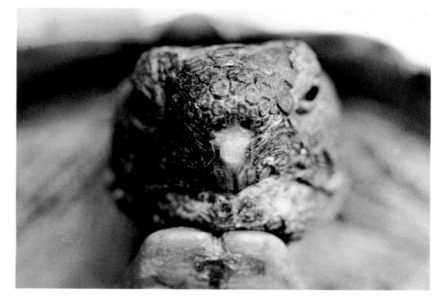

Figure 38b
Chronic respiratory infection in a gopher tortoise. Note the excoriation ventral to the nostrils.

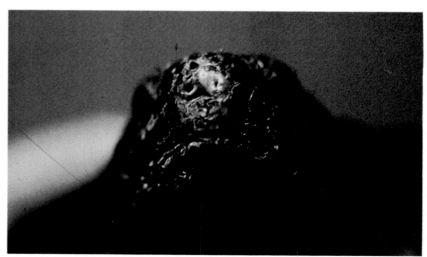

Figure 38c
Chronic respiratory infection in a desert tortoise. The nostrils are partially occluded.

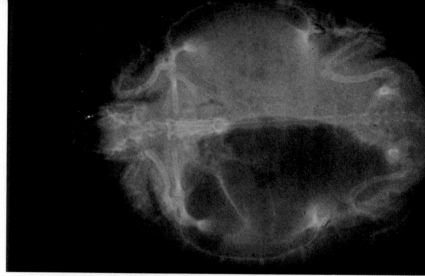

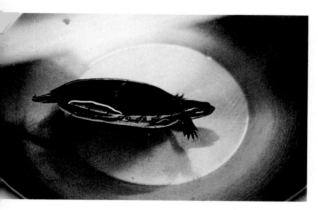

Figure 39—Swimming attitude of an aquatic turtle with a respiratory infection. An exudate-filled or collapsed lung disturbs normal hydrostatic balance.

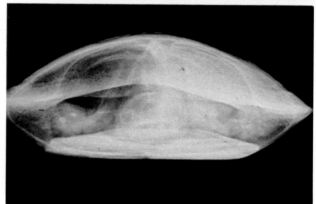

Figures 40a & 40b—Radiographs of the turtle shown in Figure 39. Note the radio-dense left side and well aerated right lung field.

B. Respiratory Infections

Respiratory infections are common in all captive species. They are of particular importance in chelonians. Signs are inappetance, torpor, nasal discharge, open-mouth breathing, and wheezing (*Figures 38a-38c*).

Occasionally, the presenting sign or complaint as described by the owner is the loss of normal swimming equilibrium. This causes the turtle to have a longitudinally slanted appearance in the tank, one side being lower than the other. Since the pulmonary system of aquatic chelonians also functions as an efficient hydrostatic organ for maintaining various states of buoyancy, a unilateral loss of the functional pulmonary bed causes the turtle to swim with a marked list. The affected, nonaerated side will be lowermost (*Figures 39, 40a & 40b, 41a-41c*).

Inspiratory effort in chelonians is mostly an active process; expiration is mostly passive. Therefore, the clearance of exudates from distal respiratory spaces is inefficient. The high incidence of respiratory disease in captive turtles and tortoises attests to the jeopardy in which these animals are placed when they are stressed sufficiently to become clinically diseased.

In the past, newly-captured tortoises have started on their journey to the pet-animal trade with few, if any, advantages. After capture, they were placed in holding cages of varying population density without regard to size, sex or state of health. Feeding, watering and sanitation were haphazard at best. That morbidity and mortality under these conditions are excessive is no wonder.

Treatment

Ampicillin or chloromycetin plus ascorbic acid is used in treatment of respiratory diseases of chelonians. Injection sites are the posterior aspect of the rear legs, and the thigh area. Intraperitoneal injection may be used

Figures 41a & 41b—Postmortem photographs of the turtle shown in Figure 39. Note the total collapse of the left lung and the normal air-filled right lung.

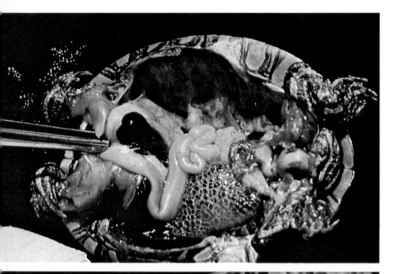

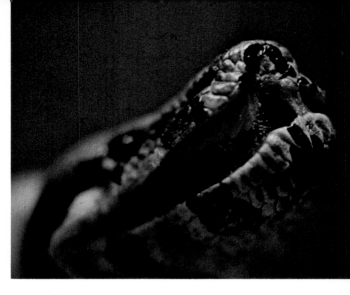

Figure 42—A boa constrictor with severe respiratory infection. Note the open-mouth breathing and thick, bubble-filled mucus.

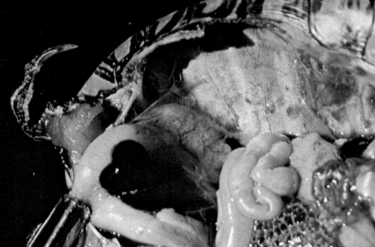

for some agents but is generally not as desirable as intramuscular injection. Husbandry practices should also be improved; most new arrivals or newly-acquired tortoises have been severely stressed from the time of their capture until they reach their ultimate destination. New arrivals should be isolated for four to six weeks before being exposed to resident specimens (*Figure 42*).

C. Infectious Stomatitis ("Mouth Rot")

Infectious stomatitis is commonly found in snakes, lizards and chelonians (*Figures 43-46*). The condition is mostly bacterial in origin,

Figure 41c
The left lung. (*See Figures 41a & 41b.*) Bronchopneumonia and atelectasis were prominent histopathologic features.

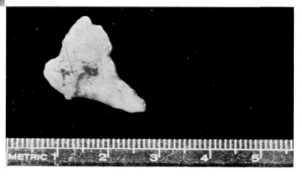

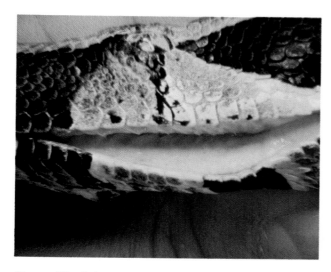

Figure 43—A boa constrictor with very early lesions of infectious stomatitis (mouth rot). Note the punctate gingival hemorrhages and excessive mucus.

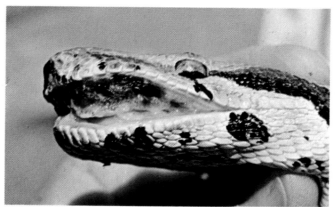

Figure 44—A more advanced case of infectious stomatitis. Invasion of subgingival tissues is evident.

with stress and poor hygiene serving as contributing factors in most cases. The etiologic agent most frequently cultured is *Aeromonas hydrophila*.

Treatment

Treatment consists of thorough cleansing of all oral tissues with hydrogen peroxide and Betadine® Solution (Purdue Frederick). Systemic antibiotics, multi-B complex vitamins and ascorbic acid are used as adjunctive therapy. Most cases respond well to ampicillin, and there is less likelihood of superinfection due to secondary opportunists when ampicillin is given. In the past, sulfamethazine and sulfaquinoxyline have also been used.

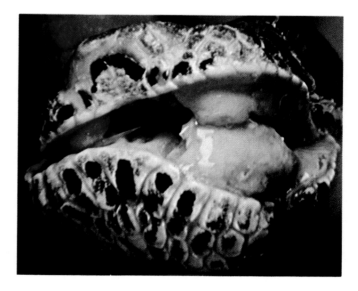

Figure 45—A very advanced case of infectious stomatitis in a boa constrictor. By this time, bone necrosis, osteomyelitis and widespread invasion of soft tissues are apparent.

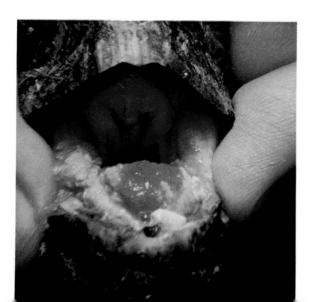

Figure 46—Infectious stomatitis in a desert tortoise. Although superficially this infection appears serious, the prognosis is good once vigorous treatment is initiated.

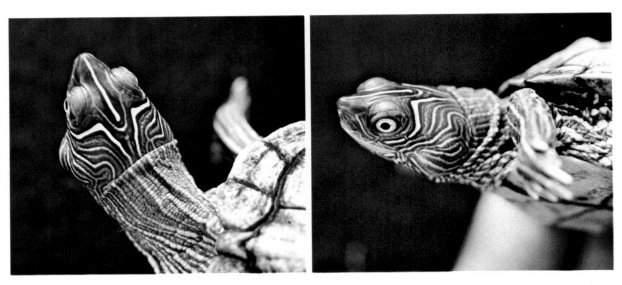

Figures 47a & 47b—A solitary abscess in the parotid region of a turtle.

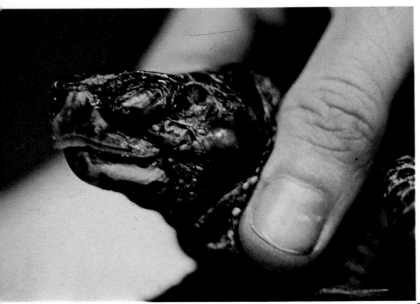

Figure 47c—A solitary abscess in the parotid region of a box tortoise.

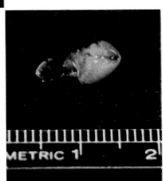

Figure 47d—Inspissated contents from the abscess seen in Figure 47c.

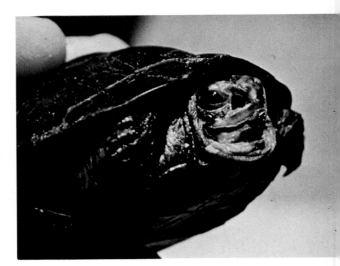

Figure 47e
Local destruction of the horn layer and underlying maxillary bone in a turtle after debridement of a single abscess. This defect was repaired with an epoxy-resin prosthesis so that the animal could feed itself more easily.

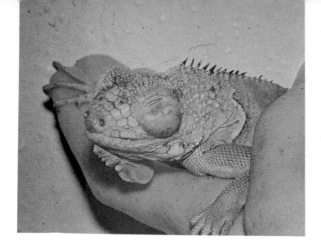

Figure 47f—Infraorbital abscess in an iguana.

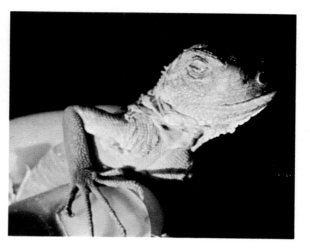

Figure 47g—Maxillary abscess in an iguana.

Figure 47h—Massive orbital abscessation in a rainbow lizard.

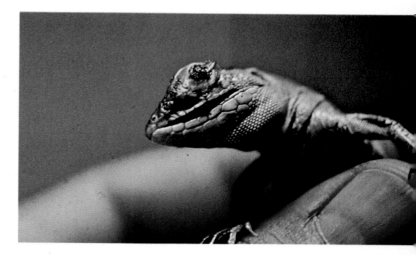

D. Abscess

Subcutaneous abscesses, common in all species, may be initiated by external wounds, parasites or hematogenous spread from a different focus (*Figures 47a-47i*). Occasionally, massive internal abscesses are encountered. Their presence should be suspected in snakes when firm swellings are palpated within the body cavity. Radiographs will show displacement of visceral organs by radiopaque densities (*Figures 48a-48c*). A stained blood film from the patient usually reveals a marked leukocytosis with eosinophilia. Snakes with such massive abscesses frequently are found to have metastatic pulmonary abscesses and purulent pericarditis (*Figure 48d*).

A number of microorganisms have been isolated from reptilian abscesses. Both pure and mixed cultures have been found. *Aeromonas, Citrobacter, Enterobacter, Escherichia, Mycobacteria, Peptostreptococcus, Proteus morganii, Proteus rettgeri, Pseudomonas, Salmonella marina* and *Serratia* have all been reported.

Obviously, some protection should be afforded the clinician when he handles patients capable of transmitting such potentially zoonotic disease organisms as those reported.

Figure 47i—Abscess of the subcorneal shield in a tree boa. This lesion was treated by incision, drainage, and flushing from beneath the orbital contents via the oral cavity.

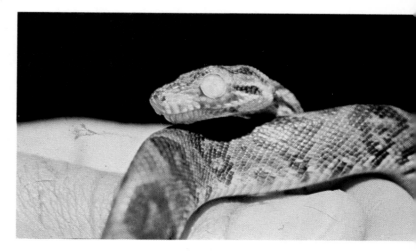

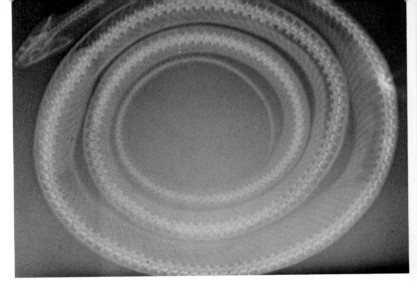

Figure 48a—A radiograph of a rat snake with massive internal abscesses. Note the three large fusiform fluid-density masses. These masses were very firm on palpation.

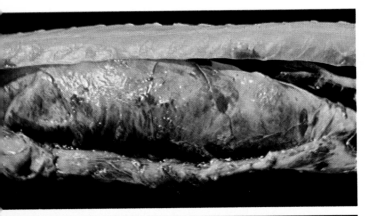

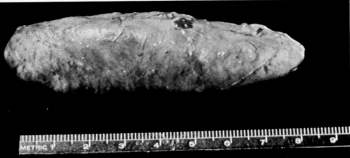

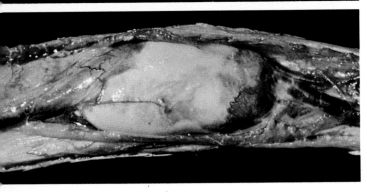

Figure 48b—One of the abscesses seen in Figure 48a, as it appeared *in situ*.

Figure 48c—One of the abscesses removed from the snake in Figure 48a. Note the well-developed capsule.

Figure 48d—Purulent pericarditis from the same rat snake (*Figures 48a-c*).

Disposable latex examination gloves are an inexpensive and effective barrier to contamination.

Quarantine of infected animals must always be strictly observed. A "clean-to-dirty" protocol should be established and maintained so that healthy animals are always handled first and no cross-contamination occurs. Thorough attention to hygiene is mandatory in this as well as other sub-specialties of veterinary medicine.

Treatment

Abscesses are treated by incision, drainage, or thorough removal of caseated debris. Anesthesia is usually not required. The abscess cavity is flushed with hydrogen peroxide (3% by volume) and Betadine Solution. The cavity can be packed with Furacin® (Eaton) and dressings can be applied if practicable.

E. Septicemic Cutaneous Ulcerative Disease (SCUD)

Septicemic cutaneous ulcerative disease is characterized in turtles by anorexia, lethargy, paralysis and cutaneous ulceration (*Figure 49*). In advanced cases, areas of necrosis are seen in visceral organs. SCUD is usually fatal if not treated. The etiologic agent has been reported to be *Citrobacter freundii*.

Treatment

Treatment consists of daily injections of Chloromycetin® succinate (Parke-Davis) in appropriate dosage.

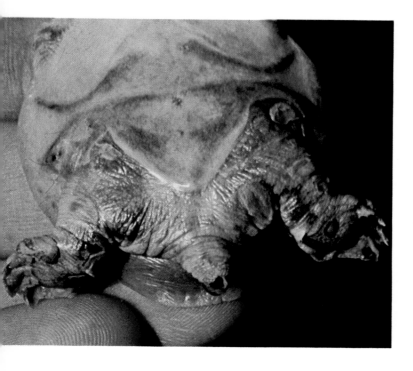

Figure 49
Septicemic cutaneous ulcerative disease (SCUD) in a soft-shelled turtle.

Figure 50a
Massive shell trauma in a gopher tortoise. Numerous fractures extend through the full thickness of both the carapace and the plastron.

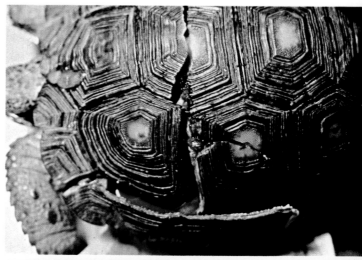

Figure 50b (below right)—A radiograph of the tortoise seen in Figure 50a.

Figure 50c (below)—Completed shell repair. An epoxy resin-impregnated fiberglass fabric was used.

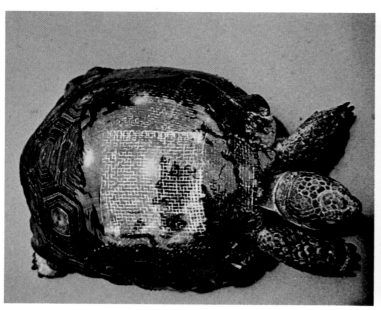

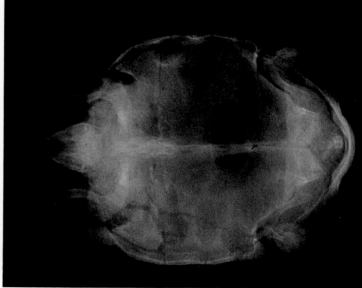

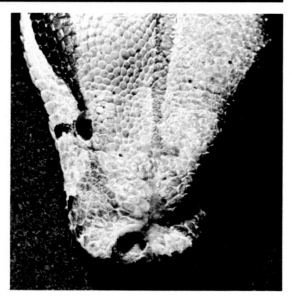

Figures 51d & 51e—Rostral abrasions in a boa constrictor and an iguana resulting from rough cage surfaces of hardware cloth.

Figures 51a to 51c—Rat-bite trauma.

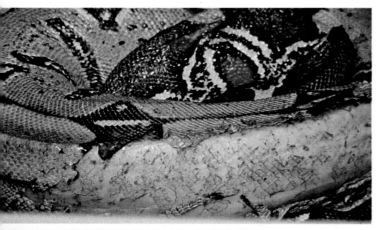

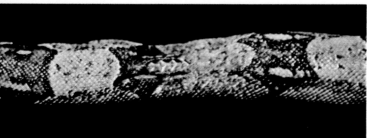

F. Trauma

The two traumatic lesions encountered most often in captive reptiles in my practice are: 1) rat bites in boas, and 2) crushing injuries in tortoises (*Figures 50a-50c*).

Rat bites can be quite serious; however, debridement and the application of Furacin on sterile dressings are usually the only treatments required. Scarring is a constant sequel since the bites usually involve the loss of much underlying soft tissue (*Figures 51a-51c*).

The problem of rat bites can be avoided by not feeding conscious live rats to snakes. Simply stunning the rats usually will eliminate the hazard of bite trauma. If the snake refuses the proffered meal, the rat is none-the-worse for wear when it awakens.

Another frequently occurring traumatic lesion is abrasion of the rostral scales and surrounding tissues in snakes which incessantly rub their snouts on wire cloth portions of their cages (*Figures 51d & 51e*). As a means of prevention, all rough surfaces—especially hardware cloth—should be removed from cages. Abraded areas should be gently cleansed and treated topically with an appropriate wound dressing, such as Furacin Ointment.

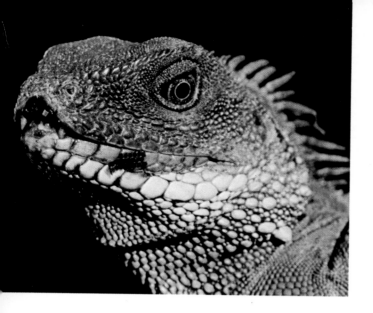

G. Thermal Burns

The use of overhead heat lamps is usually the cause of thermal burns in captive reptiles (*Figures 51f-51h, 52*).

A useful alternative to heat lamps is the employment of heating coils or thermal pads beneath the cage or litter. The resultant heat is more evenly distributed and is far safer once the heat source has been calibrated and adjusted. In small terraria, heating pads work well under a cage which has been placed on corner blocks or spacers. (*See diagram, page 19*).

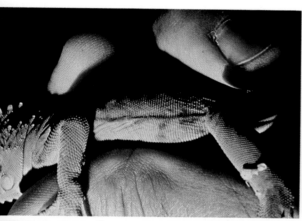

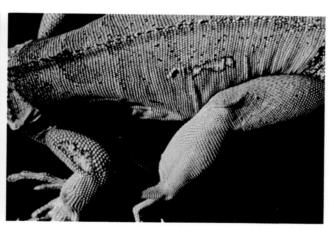

Figures 51f to 51h—Thermal burns in two iguanas and a boa constrictor.

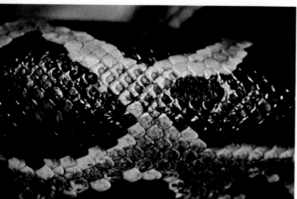

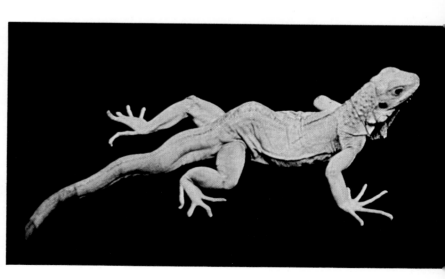

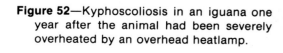

Figure 52—Kyphoscoliosis in an iguana one year after the animal had been severely overheated by an overhead heatlamp.

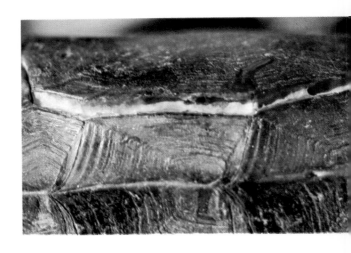

Miscellaneous
Bacterial Diseases
(*Figures 54a-54g*)

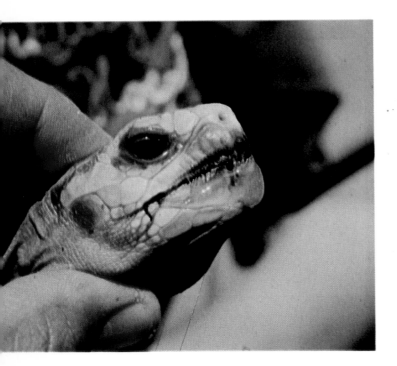

Figure 53—A small fracture of the mandibular beak repaired with rapid-polymerizing epoxy resin.

H. Shell Defects

Shell defects in chelonians are often a challenge because of their complexity, but they are always fun to treat. After the exposed soft tissues have been cleansed with tepid Ringer's solution, to which has been added Daribiotic® (Beecham-Massengill), the shreds of loose tissue and the avascular shell fragments are debrided. Debridement is followed with another lavage. All raw edges are painted with Betadine Solution, air-dried with a hand-held hair dryer, and then patched together in apposition with fiberglass fabric impregnated with epoxy resin.

We are now using a rapid polymerizing epoxy resin, Devco® 5-Minute Epoxy (Devcon Corp.), for repair of shell defects. After approximately one year, the growth areas are routed away with a hand-held rotary bit to allow for future expansion. No untoward reactions have been experienced with this material, even though there is a local temperature elevation as the polymerization reaches its peak. Apparently, polymerization time is short enough and the dissipation of the heat of reaction is adequate to prevent tissue damage. Primary healing has been achieved in every case treated.

After repair, an appropriate dosage of ampicillin trihydrate (Polyflex®—Bristol) is injected intramuscularly and repeated daily for two to five days.

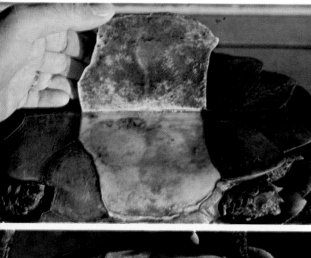

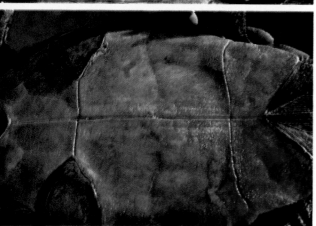

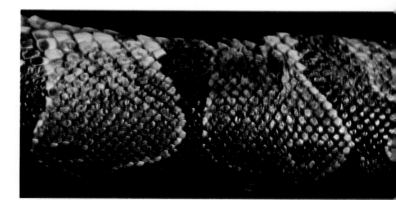

Figures 54a to 54c—Shell-plate separation in a tortoise. In severe cases the entire shellplate pattern of the plastron may be lost.

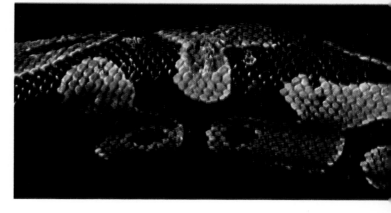

Figures 54d & 54e—Superficial dermal ulceration in two boa constrictors. Both of these snakes had been kept in overly-moist environments where sanitation was poor.

I. Shell-Plate Sloughing

Sometimes, in captive chelonians, a horny shell plate (or more than one) will be loosened from its underlying bony bed or will be found to be missing entirely (*Figures 54a-54c*). My experience suggests that the incidence of this problem is greatest in terrestrial forms kept under unsanitary conditions. Too much moisture and a buildup of fecal-borne bacteria, in already stressed animals, work synergistically to produce disease.

Treatment consists of careful cleansing of affected exposed tissue and the application of suitable antimicrobial agents. Appropriate antibiotics should be employed. It is also important that pre-existing husbandry practices be altered to reflect attention to the animal's native habitat.

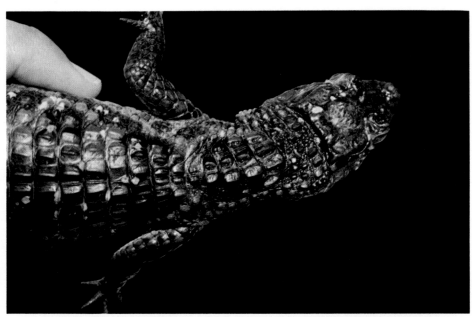

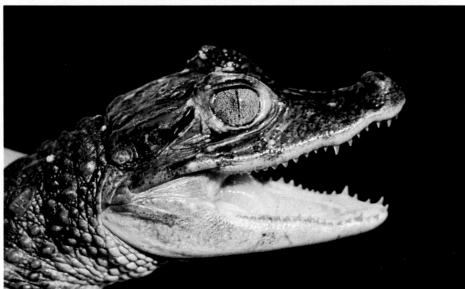

Figures 54f & 54g—Dorsal and lateral views of a baby crocodile with multiple punctate foci of superficial dermatitis. These lesions respond well to local treatment and improved sanitation procedures.

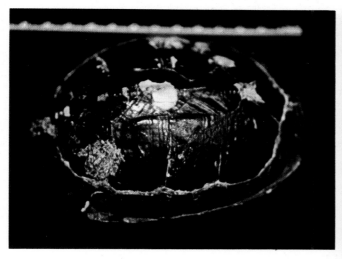

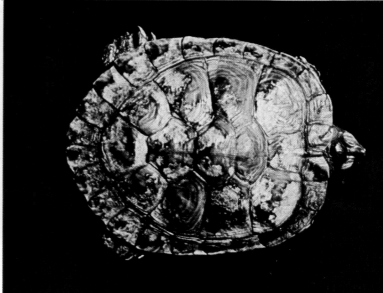

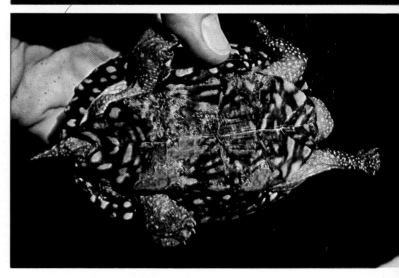

J. Shell Fungus

Shell fungus is a common disorder of aquatic chelonians. It is manifested by pitted, excoriated, pale areas of lifted shell substrate (*Figures 55a-55c*). The condition is infectious; therefore, affected individuals must be isolated.

Treatment

Treatment consists of local debridement and painting with Betadine Solution twice daily. While undergoing treatment, turtles should be kept dry, except to feed.

K. Salmonellosis

Much publicity has recently been given to the potential public health hazard in exposure to some aquatic chelonians. The genesis of this problem stems from the practice of rearing and collecting turtles in sewage-contaminated settling ponds and marshes in the southeastern United States, particularly in Louisiana, Mississippi and Alabama.

Another source of infection in these turtles results from the practice of feeding slaughterhouse offal, condemned carcasses, and other waste materials to the feral breeding population. These feed items frequently are heavily contaminated by *Salmonella* and *Arizona* organisms.

Figures 55a to 55c—Lesions of shell fungus in three turtles. Note the loss of the superficial horny shell layers.

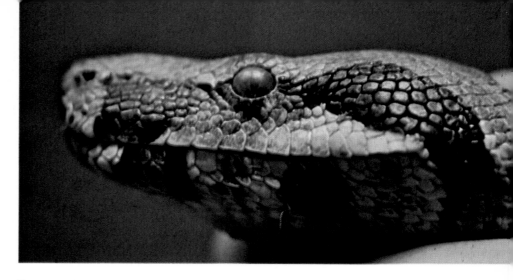

Figures 56a & 56b—Pre-ecdysis corneal opacity. The eyes have a cloudy appearance. This is a normal preshedding phenomenon.

The State of California has taken an immense stride in controlling the distribution of pet turtles by adopting regulations aimed at reducing the significant health hazard potential in these animals. These regulations are included in this text to serve as a model. (*See facing page.*)

Although attempts to certify breeding environments free of *Salmonella* and *Arizona* organisms are being made, it is an almost impossible task since many nonpathogenic forms of these two genera are commonly found among the gastrointestinal microflora of aquatic chelonians. Also, the opportunity for environmental contamination from wildlife is always present.

Carrier turtles do not generally exhibit any observable signs of salmonella infection. Positive salmonella isolations are made from stool cultures or pooled cultures from water in which the turtles have been kept.

Treatment

Treatment is accomplished by the use of appropriate antibiotics. Chloromycetin, neomycin sulfate, and Furoxone® (Eaton) have been used with some success. However, pre-vention is much less expensive and more practical. Routine hygiene, such as hand-washing after handling, would appear to be the ideal prophylaxis.

The exclusion of turtles from the menageries of the very young would seem desirable from two standpoints. First, the incidence of turtle-associated salmonellosis in children would be reduced greatly. Secondly, the dismal situation of very short lifespans of "dimestore" turtles could be ameliorated. We know that the longevity of such turtles is proportional to the age of the principal owner.

L. Dysecdysis

Impaired skin-shedding is a common problem in captive reptiles, particularly snakes. In the normal course of events, a snake will refuse food seven to ten days before shedding. The eyes become progressively dull and eventually appear to be covered with an opaque, bluish-white corneal film (*Figures 56a & 56b*). This opacity soon fades. At the same time, the skin coloration becomes dull. These changes are the result of oil secretion between the old and underlying healthy epidermis.

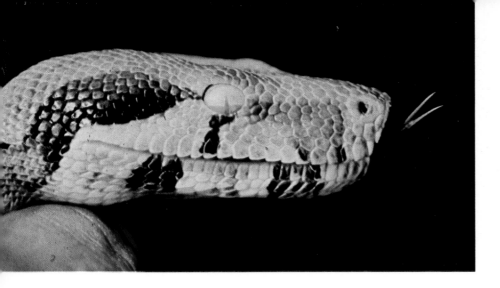

REGULATIONS GOVERNING THE IMPORTATION, SALE AND DISTRIBUTION OF LIVE TURTLES IN CALIFORNIA

Section 2612.1, Title 17, California Administrative Code

(a) It shall be unlawful to import, sell or offer for sale or distribution to the public a live turtle unless such turtle(s) are certified to be free from *Salmonella* and *Arizona* organisms. The certifying authority and the method used to determine freedom from *Salmonella* and *Arizona* organisms for shipment of turtles into and for offering for sale within California must be acceptable to and be approved by the Department before being shipped into the State.

(b) All persons selling or offering for sale or distribution turtles at wholesale shall provide the retailer with a written statement of approved certification of freedom from *Salmonella* and *Arizona* organisms for each lot of turtles.

(c) The State Department of Public Health or any authorized representative thereof, or any local health officer or his representative may quarantine turtles, take samples of tank water or any other appropriate samples of or from turtles offered for sale or distribution for the purpose of testing for *Salmonella* and *Arizona* organisms. The Department or any local health officer shall order the immediate humane destruction of any lot of turtles found contaminated with *Salmonella, Arizona,* or other organisms which may cause disease in humans. humans.

(d) Shipments of turtles may be authorized by the Department in writing to a governmental agency, or to recognized research institutions or zoological gardens for display or research purposes provided the turtles or the environment where the turtles are to be kept shall not constitute a hazard to the public. All such requests must be made to the Department in writing.

(e) The following warning must be posted conspicuously for buyer information at every display of turtles for retail sale or distribution or where the public may come in contact with turtles:

> CAUTION: Turtles may transmit bacteria causing disease in humans. It is important to wash the hands thoroughly after handling turtles or material in a turtle bowl. Do not allow water or any other substance from a turtle bowl to come in contact with food or areas where food is prepared. Make sure that these precautions are followed by children and others handling turtles.

(f) For each sale of turtle(s) at retail, a sales slip shall be issued by the seller to the purchaser at time of the sale. The sales slip shall include the name, address and telephone number of the purchaser and the seller, and the date of sale. The sales slip shall have printed legibly on its front the warning statement contained in subsection (e) above. The seller shall keep a copy of the sales slip, which shall include the name, address and telephone number of the purchaser for not less than one year, and keep a complete record of all purchases, losses and other dispositions of turtles.

Effective date November 4, 1972

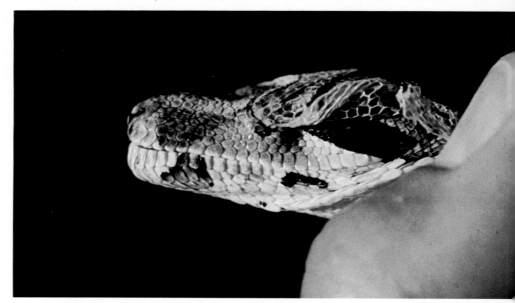

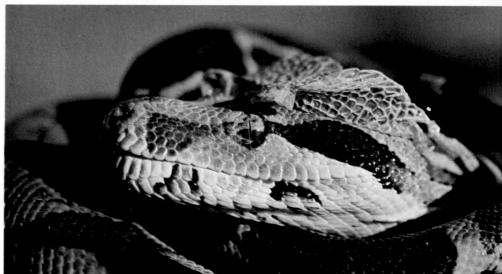

Figures 57a & 57b
Progression of shedding
eyecaps (spectacles).

Figures 57c & 57d—Intact skin from an indigo snake (*Drymarchon corais*). The spectacles, which normally are shed each time the outer skin layers are renewed, are intact.

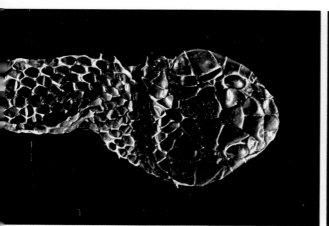

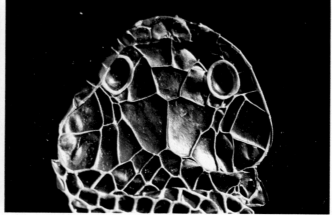

In order to shed, the snake rubs its chin and nose on environmental surfaces until the outer senescent skin at the mucocutaneous junction of the mouth is loosened sufficiently to separate from the underlying living epidermal tissues. The snake now actively crawls from the outer covering, usually turning it inside out in the process (*Figures 57a-57d*). Rough surfaces such as logs, branches, forest litter, etc. aid in the process.

If a snake is dehydrated or otherwise debilitated, the process of shedding may be impaired or delayed (*Figure 58*). Soaking the snake in tepid water and then sandwiching it between moistened toweling aids greatly in the removal of dried, non-separated skin. Gentle help with a washcloth may also be required. An adequate water supply and cage enrichment, such as logs and branches, are essential.

Occasionally, a snake will shed its skin properly, but will fail to shed one or both of the corneal shields (*Figure 59*). These shields can be removed easily by gentle lifting and traction with a fine forceps. If the shields do not part with relative ease, the application of warm, moist compresses will aid further in their removal. Force must not be used, as the corneas can be irreparably damaged by traumatic avulsion of dry, adherent shields (*Figure 60*).

Dysecdysis (*Figures 58 & 59*)

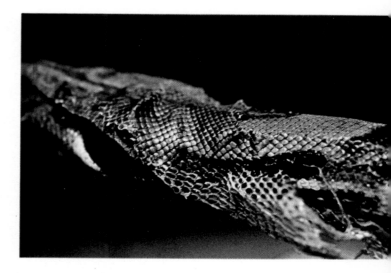

Figure 58
Failure to shed the skin in a single piece. The remnants soon dry and become adherent.

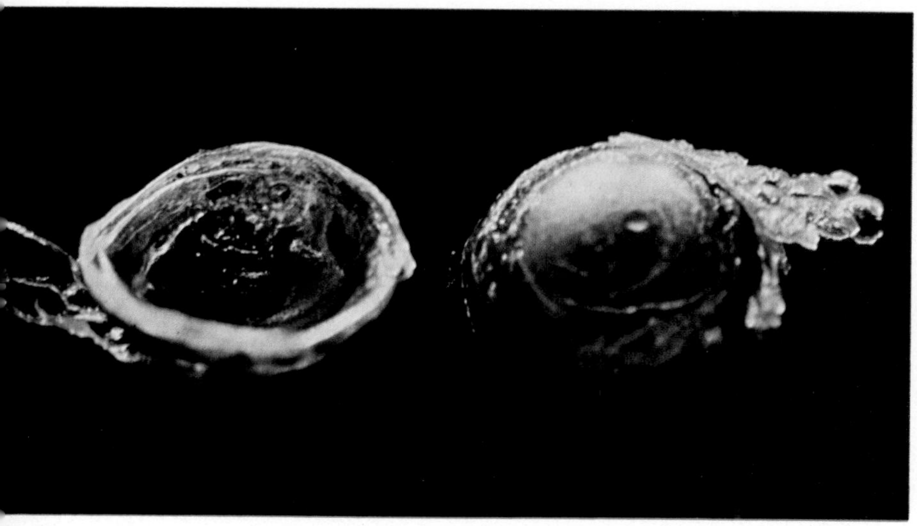

Figure 59
Multilayered spectacles from a snake which had failed to shed normally through several molts.

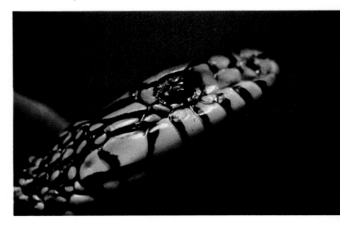

Figure 60—Cornea of a snake showing trauma resulting from forced avulsion of dry retained spectacles.

M. Fluid Replacement Therapy

Subcutaneous or intraperitoneal infusion is indicated for patients in which clinical dehydration is detected or suspected.

A modified reptilian Ringer's solution has been found to be accepted well by reptiles. The formula is adapted from one designed to be isotonic with respect to the cerebrospinal fluid of some turtles (Fleisey, S.R.: *Federation Proceedings 27*:287; 1968). The composition of the medium, per 1000 cc. of sterile water for injection:

> Sodium . . . . 128 mEq.
> Potassium . . . . 2.6 mEq.
> Calcium . . . . 2 mEq.
> Magnesium . . . . 2 mEq.
> Chloride . . . . 112 mEq.
> Bicarbonate . . . . 20 mEq.

The volume administered is determined according to the relative degree of dehydration. If desired, glucose and vitamins may be added to the solution.

N. Ophthalmic Diseases

Probably the most frequently encountered eye problem in captive reptiles, particularly snakes and lizards, is panophthalmitis with orbital abscessation (*Figures 61, 47i*). Even when at first inspection the eye appears to be completely obliterated, incision and drainage from beneath the orbital tissues may result in a return to full function. Snakes commonly are presented with one or both eyes completely invisible beneath purulent exudate.

Treatment

A small incision, either via the oral cavity or immediately beneath the corneal shield, will provide access to the site of the retrocorneal shield. Inspissated pus and cellular detritus can be removed gently with a smooth probe or flattened curette. Flushing with Ringer's solution, to which neomycin sulfate solution has been added, aids in removing any residual debris. Parenteral antibiotic coverage should also be provided.

Common Eye Lesions (*Figures 60-63*)

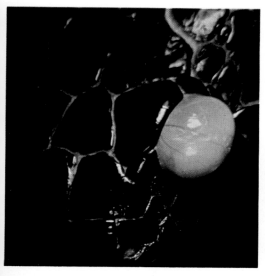

Figure 61—Panophthalmitis in an indigo snake (*Drymarchon corais*). The affected eye and its adnexa were enucleated.

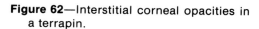
Figure 62—Interstitial corneal opacities in a terrapin.

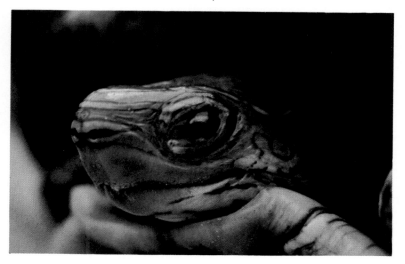

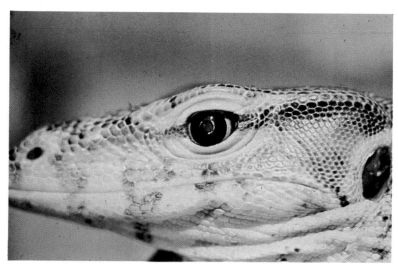

Figure 63—Lenticular opacities in a monitor lizard. There was no apparent visual deficit in this animal.

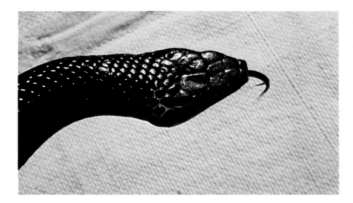

Figure 64a
Firm swelling of the parotid area in an indigo snake.

Figure 64b
An impression smear from
the lesion seen in the snake
in Figure 64a (Giemsa x 320).

Figure 64c
A histopathologic section.
Marked eosinophilia char-
acterizes this verminous
granuloma. Note the num-
erous well-defined eosinophils (H & E x 430).

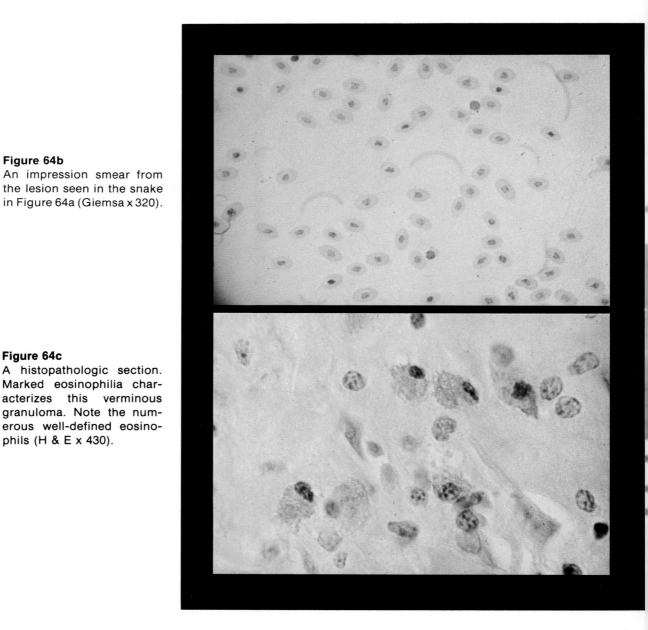

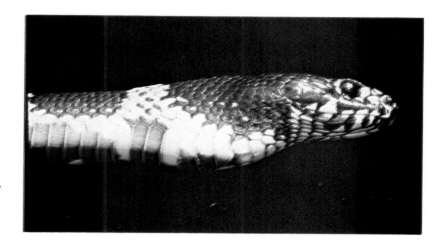

Figure 64d
Intermandibular and ventral cervical mass in a California king snake (*Lampropeltis getulus californiae*).

O. Pseudoneoplasms

Pseudoneoplasms are firm-to-fluctuant swellings most frequently found in terrestial snakes. I have excised several from different species of common North American snakes. In every case, helminth parasites, hemogregarines and trypanosomes were found in mixed infections (*Figures 64a-64m, 65a-65c*).

Histopathologically, these lesions represent eosinophilic granulomata and verminous cysts. Prior to specific treatment, stained impression smears should be examined for the etiologic agent(s). Treatment consists of thorough excision, debridement, and packing with an appropriate medication (such as povidone-impregnated gauze sponge, mild silver nitrate, 4% buffered formalin, etc.).

These pseudoneoplasms are characteristically very vascular and they bleed excessively. Hemorrhage can be controlled by pressure or pinpoint electrocautery. After debridement and hemostasis have been accomplished, dead space is obliterated and skin edges are sutured with nonabsorbable suture material.

Mycotic granulomata occasionally occur in reptiles. These lesions may be firm, nonyielding swellings resembling subcutaneous abscesses; or they may appear as soft, semifluctuant blebs loosely covered with normal skin. The latter type of lesion is found more frequently in lizards, especially the American anole (*Figure 65a*).

Stained impression smears should be employed to establish the definitive diagnosis.

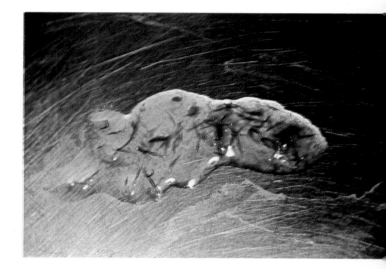

Figure 64e
Gross appearance of the exudate (lesion shown in Figure 64d).

Pseudoneoplasms

Figures 64f to 64i—Stained impression smears. (*See Figures 64d & 64e.*) Hemogregarines, trypanosomes and microfilariae were recovered from the exudate.

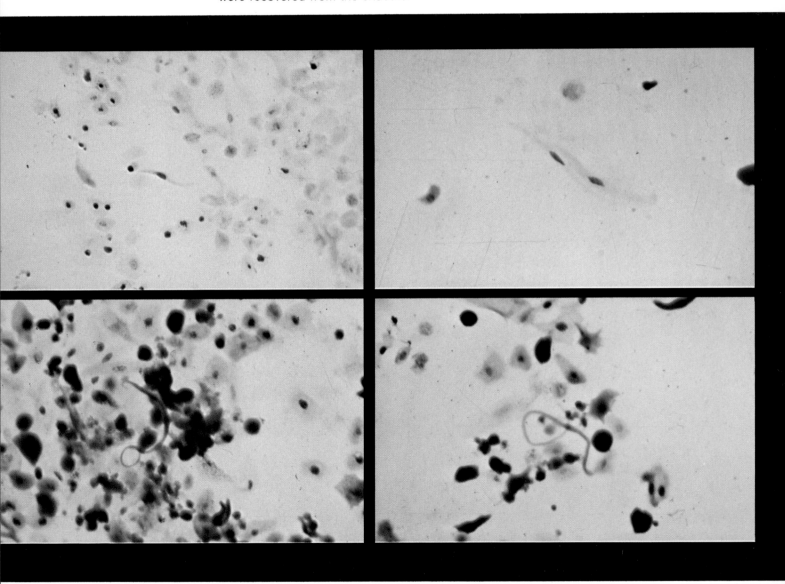

Figure 64j—A pseudoneoplasm between the right nostril and lip in an iguana. Note the ulcerated surface.

Figures 64k & 64l—Histopathologic sections of the lesion seen in Figure 64j. Pathologic diagnosis was foreign body (verminous) granuloma and inclusion cyst (H & E x 100).

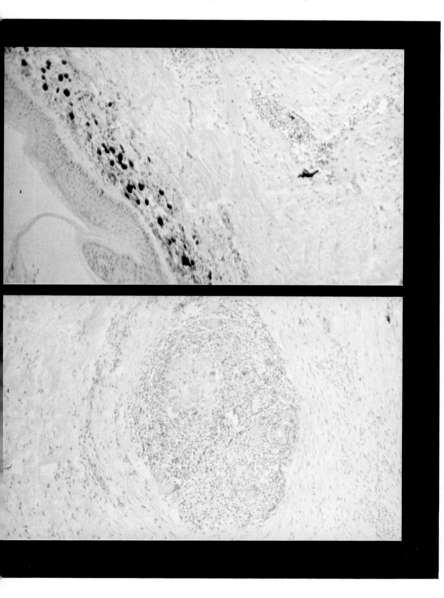

Figure 64m—A pseudoneoplasm involving the lower-left rear leg of an *Uromastix hardwickii*. The lesion was removed surgically and found to be a chronic granuloma.

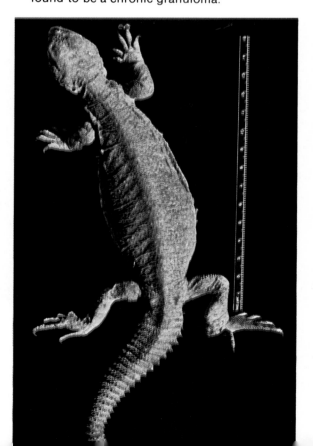

Pseudoneoplasms

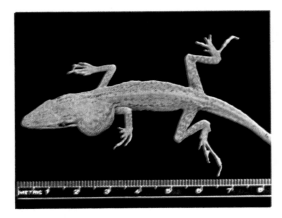

Figure 65a—A large fluctuant mass in an American anole. After removal of the mass, impression smears and tissue sections were made.

Figures 65b & 65c—These are stained impression smears. (*See Figure 65a.*) Note the refractile macroconidia among cellular debris and engulfed within a macrophage. The diagnosis was organizing hematoma and mycotic granuloma (Giemsa x 680).

Refractile mycelia or macroconidia are seen in smears from these lesions (*Figures 65b & 65c*).

Treatment consists of wide excision, curettage and appropriate packing of the wound—with or without suturing, depending on location, tissue loss, etc.

In the single case which I have had the opportunity to examine, subcutaneous masses, which appeared superficially to be abscesses, were found to be masses of egg-containing cestodes (*Figures 66a-66d*). The taxonomic diagnosis of this tapeworm is still much in question. This particular snake, a watersnake (*Natrix* sp.) from southeastern Europe, had been purchased from an animal exporter who could furnish no collection data. The snake was sacrificed and found to be harboring more than three hundred of these interesting tapeworms beneath its skin. No gross evidence of intestinal cestode parasitism was found on postmortem examination of the cadaver.

Preliminary study of these cestodes indicates that they are spargana or immature forms of a *Spirometra* species, perhaps *S. erinaceae europiae*. A variety of small carnivores has been fed worms recovered from this snake and attempts will be made to recover mature tapeworms from these definitive hosts. The results will be reported in the literature.

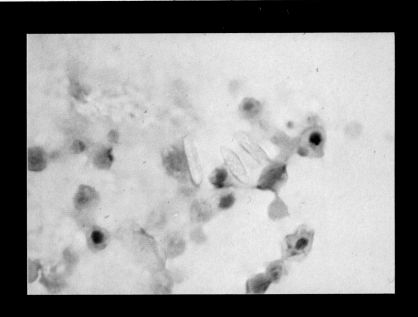

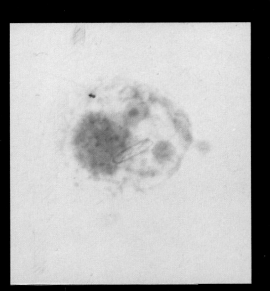

Subcutaneous Parasitism Involving Immature Cestodes (*Figures 66a-66d*)

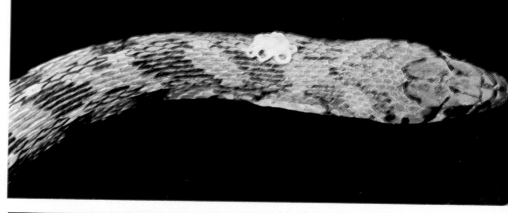

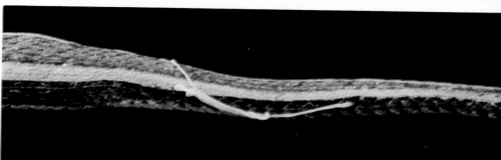

Figure 66b—Several tapeworms (*Spirometra* sp.) of the sparganum, or plerocercoid, form emerging through a small skin incision in the snake shown in Figure 66a.

Figure 66c—More than 300 individual immature worms were removed from this watersnake.

Figure 66d—Microscopic detail of the scolex. The mouthparts are simple, lacking suckers and hooklets.

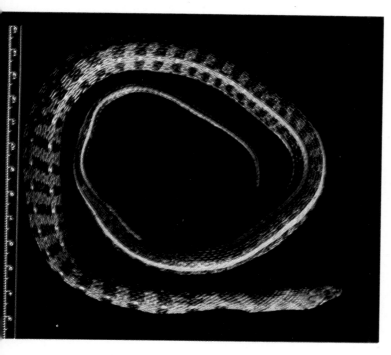

Figure 66a—Gross appearance of a watersnake (*Natrix* sp.) prior to removal of worms. Note the almost gravid appearance of the snake.

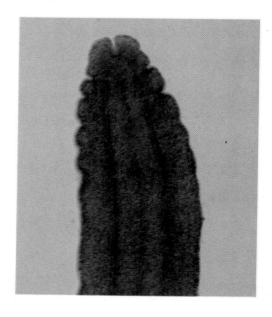

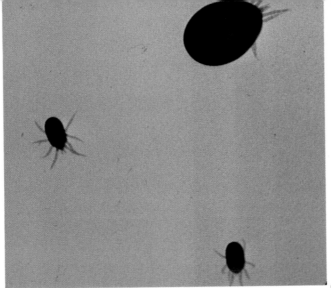

Figure 67a & 67b—Mites (*Ophionyssus natricis*); larvae and adults.

Figure 67c—A snake tick.

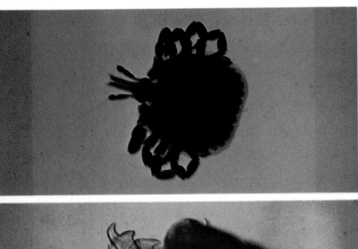

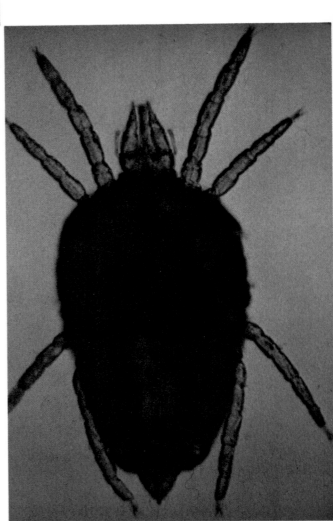

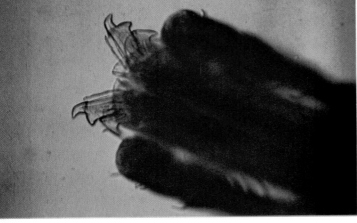

Figure 67d—Mouthparts of the tick seen in Figure 67c. The recurved hooks aid greatly in keeping the parasite attached to the host during feeding.

P. Parasitism

1. Ectoparasites

Lizards and snakes quite frequently carry ectoparasites. Mites (particularly *Ophionyssus natricis*) (*Figures 67a & 67b*) and ticks—especially *Ornithodoros* sp. (*Figures 67c & 67d*) commonly are a problem in reptile collections. Both of these arthropods have been implicated in the transmission of infectious diseases of reptiles.

The simplest measure for eradicating mites and ticks is to suspend small portions of a dichlorvos-impregnated plastic pest strip (Shell Chemical Co.) above the cage. This technique has been used with excellent effect in many collections of captive reptiles. At Steinhart Aquarium, entire pest strips have been suspended in cage rooms. Since instituting this measure, mite infestation has been eliminated to a large degree.

Soaking individual specimens in tepid water contained in appropriate vessels has also been successful. Because of the deleterious long-term pulmonary effects from repeated inhalation exposures, the use of silica aerogel products is no longer advised.

Myiasis with the larvae of *Cuterebra*, *Callitroga*, *Sarcophaga*, and other screw- and flesh-flies is also seen (*Figures 67e & 67f*). Removal, debridement and local wound treatment are usually sufficient to bring about healing.

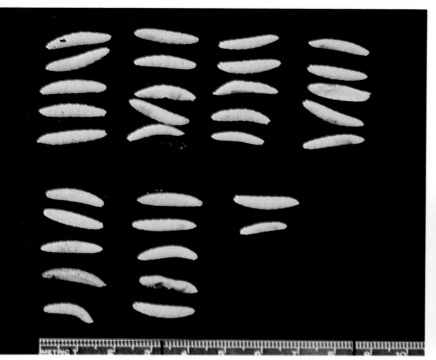

Figure 67e—Flesh-fly maggots recovered from a single three-toed box tortoise.

Figure 67f—Enlarged photograph of a single maggot. (*See Figure 67e.*)

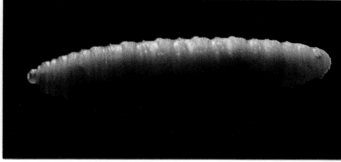

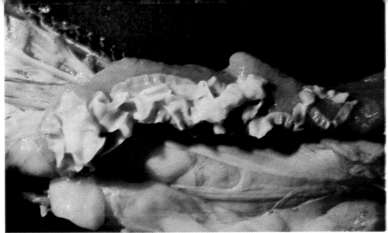

Figure 67g
Cestodes from the duodenum of a boa constrictor.

Figure 67h
Two nematodes seen through the wall of the large intestine of an iguana.

Figure 67i
Tongue worms (actually degenerate arachnids found in the upper respiratory system of a python). These parasites are transmissible to man via ingestion of infective eggs.

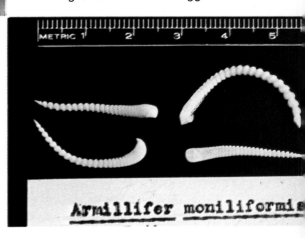

Armillifer moniliformis

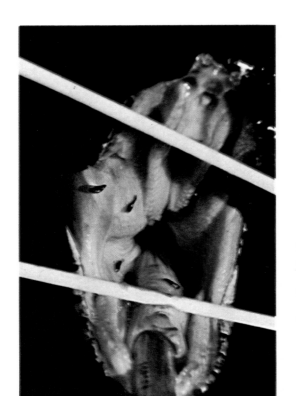

Figure 67j
Flukes of the family *Ochetosomatidae* in the oral cavity of a Florida indigo snake. Eighty-six of these flukes were recovered from this apparently healthy snake.

84

2. Endoparasites

a. Rhizopoda

Endamoeba invadens is the causative agent in reptilian ulcerative gastritis, enteritis and hepatitis. Snakes experimentally infected with cysts recovered from naturally-infected snakes became anorectic, lethargic, lost weight and began to pass blood-tinged mucus containing both cysts and trophozoites. Survival times varied between 13 and 77 days, depending on the number of cysts that had been fed.

Stomach, large and small intestine and liver are most frequently involved in amebiasis. Spread within the host is apparently via the blood and lymph vessels. Ulcers and necrosis are commonly observed. Massive hepatic necrosis may occur if hepatic portal venous branches are obstructed by thromboemboli.

Renal necrosis has been also reported to be caused by *E. invadens.*

Treatment

Intramuscular injections of emetine hydrochloride (Eli Lilly) at a dosage of 0.5 mg./kg. may be given daily for ten days. Hydration of the patient must be maintained at all times to prevent excessive serum levels due to hemoconcentration.

b. Mastigophora

Hemoflagellates, especially *Trypanosoma butananense, T. erythrolampi, T. mattogrossense* and *T. merremi,* have been found in some South American snakes. *T. sirtalis* has been observed in the North American garter snake (*Thamnophis sirtalis*). In the latter case, clinical disease was absent.

I recently recovered an unclassified trypanosome from a ventral cervical cyst in a California kingsnake (*Lampropeltis getulus californiae*). Microfilariae were found in addition to the trypanosomes. All attempts at more definitive identification of these parasites have failed (*Figures 64f-64i*).

Other hemoflagellates which reportedly have been found in clinically healthy snakes are *Herpetomonas homalosoma* var., *Eutrichomastix serpentis, Chilomastix* sp., *Trichomonas* sp. and *Giardia* sp.

c. Sporozoa

1) Coccidial infections of the gall bladder with *Eimeria bitis* have been reported. The gall bladder mucosa was found to be severely damaged and the bile was quite viscid.

Isospora naiae has also been reported to produce gall bladder and intestinal pathology.

Treatment

Sulfamethazine or sulfadimethoxine at the appropriate dosage should be instituted as soon as positive diagnosis is made from stool specimens. (*See drug dosage table, page 105.*)

2) Sporozoan parasites of the genus *Haemogregarina* are frequently seen in snake blood (*Figures 68a & 68b*). There are many species within the genus.

In one report of *H. serpentina* infection, the parasite was found in association with the linguatulid arthropod *Armillifer moniliformis.* The possibility exists that the *Armillifer* may have been the original host.

As yet, *Haemogregarina* has not been proved to be implicated in clinical disease in snakes.

d. Metazoan Parasites

Nematodes, cestodes and trematodes have all been found in reptiles. Since the diet of most snakes consists of living animals of many different species which serve as intermediate hosts for these parasites, exposure of the snakes is assured (*Figures 67g & 67h*).

Linguatuliasis is a common finding in snakes. A number of "tongue worms" (degenerate, legless parasites) infect snakes (*Figure 67i*). Generally, linguatulids pass

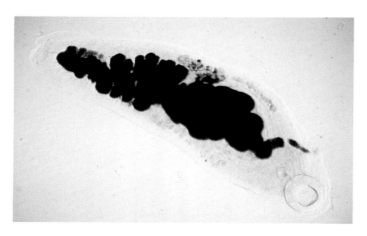

Figure 67k—A cleared specimen from Figure 64h (unstained x 10).

through an egg-to-larval stage in one host and through nymphal and adult stages in another. Most commonly, a fish or mammal is the intermediate host. After completing its migration, the mature *Armillifer* destroys pulmonary tissue. Cysts are passed via the sputum of the infected snake.

To avoid cross-contamination via water bowls, cages, caretakers' hands, etc., careful attention must be given to hygiene. No effective treatment is known. Recognized carriers should be either isolated or destroyed.

Porocephalus crotali is a related linguatulid frequently found in rattlesnakes.

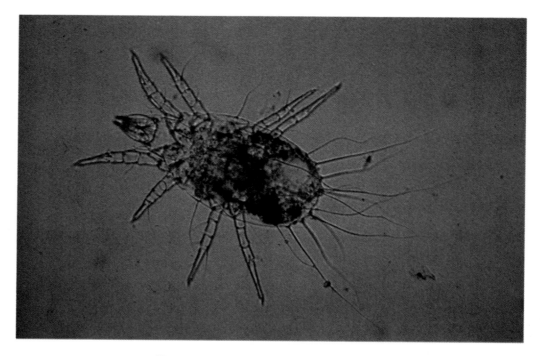

Figure 67l—Grain mite. This is not an obligatory parasite, but it may be present in large numbers in litter material.

3. Treatment for Nematode and Cestode Infestations

Treatment for specific parasite infestations is both possible and desirable. There are myriads of both cestode and nematode parasites which infest reptiles. The purpose of this text is best served by stating only that the reptiles represent a wide spectrum of hosts for many helminths. Niclosamide (Yomesan®—Chemagro) is effective against cestodes when the dosage is tailored to the bodyweight and physical condition of the patient. Both piperazine citrate and thiabendazole (Thibenzole®—Merck) have been used successfully for nematode parasites. If thiabendazole, a very hydroscopic compound, is to be given, it should first be premixed to the point that the addition of more water to the final dilution will not cause further expansion in volume. Failure to observe this precaution may result in gastrointestinal impaction or fluid and electrolyte shifts, with fatal results.

Vermifuges are most easily administered via stomach tube wherever possible.

4. Trematode Infestations

A number of species of flukes are found in almost all captive, wild-bred reptiles. While most of these trematodes will be found at necropsy, some are easily seen on physical examination of the oropharynx or eyes.

The flukes most commonly seen in reptiles belong to the family *Ochetosomatidae*. These are often found in the respiratory and upper digestive tracts of snakes (*Figures 67j & 67k*).

The life cycle of the flukes usually involves eggs being passed in the feces of the host. These eggs soon hatch after being ingested by an aquatic snail. Xiphidcocercariae of the armatae group develop in daughter sporocysts. Upon leaving the snail, the cercariae penetrates and encysts in tadpoles, particularly the genera *Rana* and *Hyla*. Infected tadpoles are eaten by a snake. Mature flukes can be found in the oropharynx and esophagus of the snake about 35 days after the metacercariae have been ingested.

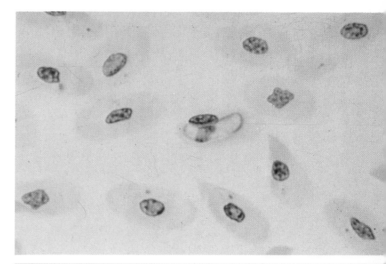

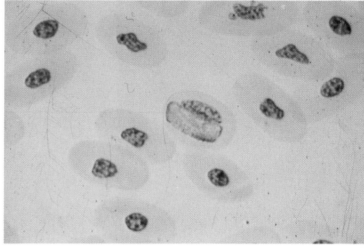

Figures 68a & 68b—Hemogregarine parasites (*Hepatazoon rarefaciens*) from a boa constrictor.

Developmental Anomalies (*Figures 69a-69e*)

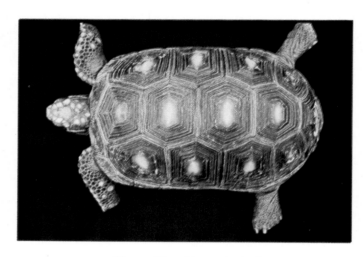

Figure 69a—Normal shell pattern in the South American redfooted tortoise.

Q. Anomalies

Congenital or heritable malformations have been seen in almost all reptilian species. The San Diego Zoo has for many years displayed specimens of two-headed snakes, albino snakes, many-tailed lizards, etc. Occasionally, a two-headed turtle or snake will be presented for examination. Almost invariably, one head will be dominant over its twin.

The most common developmental anomaly seen in captive reptile practice is the presence of asymmetrical shell defects in chelonians. These are usually wedge-shaped plates staggered neatly down the dorsal midline of the tortoises' carapaces (*Figures 69a-69e*). Apparently, these defects are completely benign and are of academic interest only.

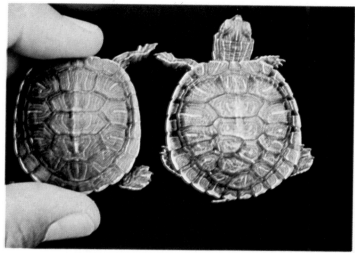

Figure 69d—Normal and asymmetrical patterns in the carapace of a *Pseudemys scripta elegans.*

Figure 69b—Anomalous asymmetrical shell-plate pattern in a South American redfooted tortoise.

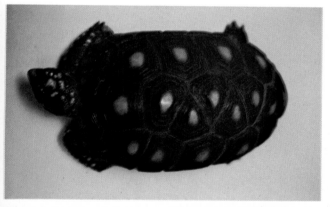

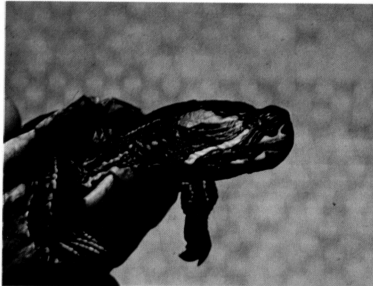

Figure 69e—Anophthalmia in a *Pseudemys scripta elegans.*

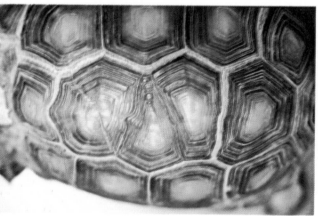

Figure 69c—Irregular shell pattern in a gopher tortoise.

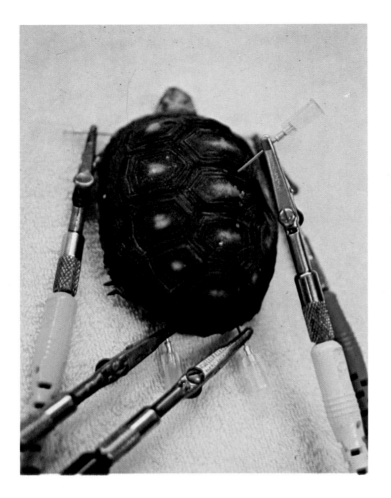

Figure 70
Placement of electrodes in a tortoise. The usual four-limb lead technique, with or without a central control lead, is satisfactory.

Figure 71
Cathode-ray tube display may be used to monitor the patient during surgery.

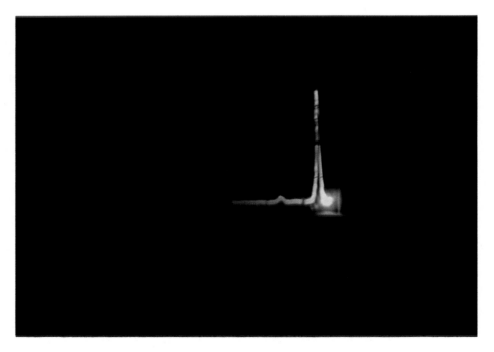

R. Radiology

Both screen and non-screen films and the respective techniques are employed in radiologic diagnosis relative to reptile medicine and surgery. Kodak's Redi-Pak® non-screen film is used most frequently. A constant technique of 125 ma., 1/6 second, and 21 Ma.S. is employed; only the kvp. is varied according to the depth of the subject and the presence of bony armor plates or scales. If faster exposure times are required, high-speed screen film in high-speed cassettes may be used with a correspondingly appropriate radiographic technique.

A word of caution: If an active, heavy tortoise is placed on the Redi-Pak® film envelope and allowed to walk across it while in contact with the pack, scratch marks will invariably appear as artifacts on the emulsion. In such a case, high-speed screen film in a cassette is more practical.

If lateral views of chelonians are desired, Ivalon® polyurethane foam bolsters should be used to position and hold the patient during the exposure. The foam is radiolucent. If necessary, the patient can be taped in position while the exposure is being made.

S. Cardiology

While still very much in its infancy, electrocardiology as an aid to diagnoses of diseased states in reptiles should be given some recognition.

Until additional normal and pathologic examples can be obtained for comparative study, only the most meager descriptions can be offered. Perhaps this lack will motivate others to explore this almost virgin field.

Standard limb leads, plus a centrally-placed control lead, are employed. Sensitivity may be 0.5, 1.0, or 1.5 millivolts, depending on the individual patient. Because all reptiles have a relatively slow heart rate, a paper speed of 25 will suffice for most specimens.

Placement of electrodes is best accomplished by using needle electrodes; sterile, disposable 20-gauge hypodermic needles with stainless steel cannulae and plastic Luer hubs work well for this purpose. The needles are firmly grasped with alligator clips attached to the lead terminals (*Figures 70 & 71*). For use with chelonian patients, the central control electrode may have to be inserted through a small hole drilled through the carapace. Later this tiny hole can be filled with epoxy resin.

The electrodes are placed on both right- and left-side locations on snakes, at the approximate sites where the fore and hind legs would be if snakes had such appendages.

Surprisingly, most reptiles will tolerate the manipulations associated with obtaining good electrocardiographic tracings. Gentle digital pressure over the eyes produces a marked calming effect in crocodilia and some lizards. Following release of this mild pressure, the animal will often remain quiet for several minutes; the tracings may then be made.

Figures 72-77 illustrate both normal and pathologic electrographic tracings.

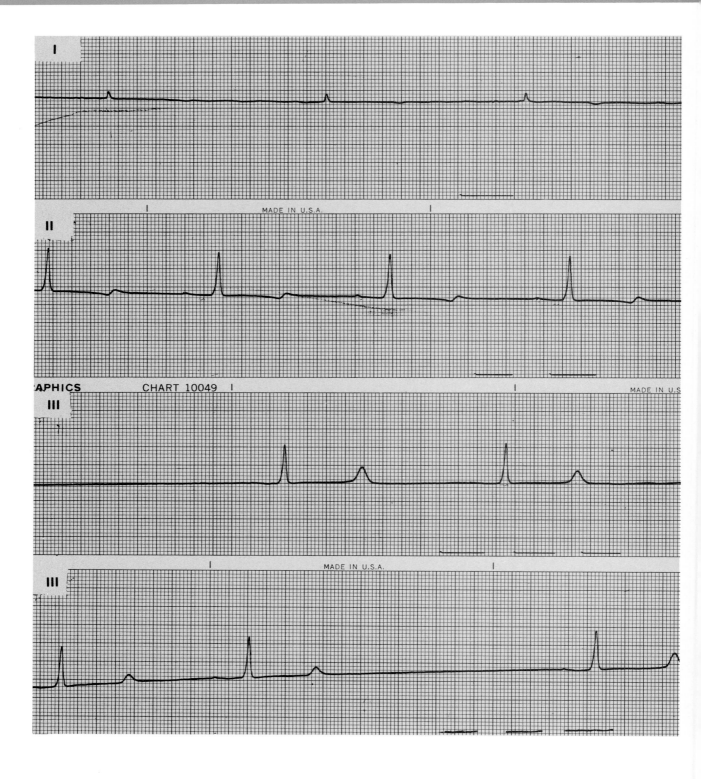

I

II

CHART 10049

III

III

MADE IN U.S.A.

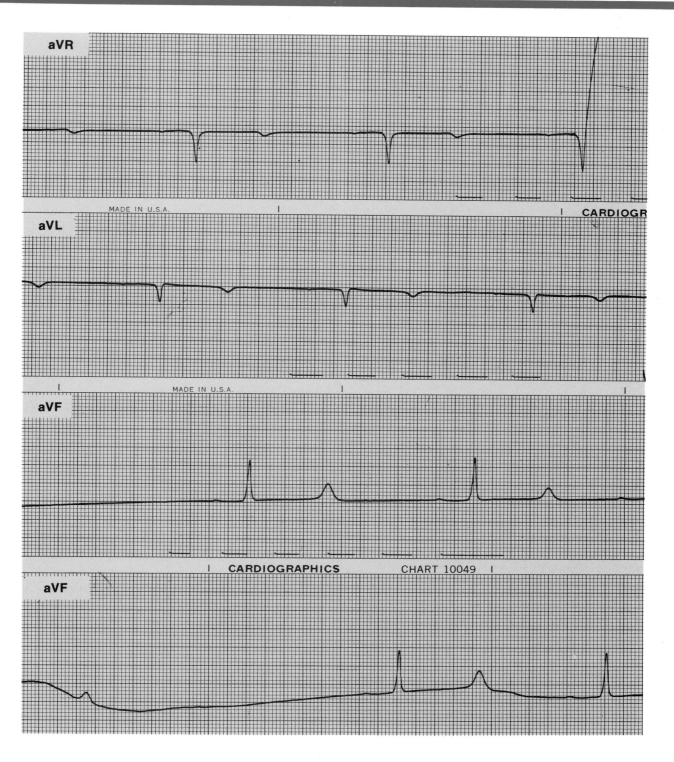

Figure 72
Clinically normal adult female redfooted tortoise (*Geochelone carbonaria*).

Ventricular rate........ approximately 40/minute	R-wave amplitude .... 1.1 millivolts
P-R interval .... 0.30 second	Electrical axis .... approximately 70°
Q-R-S interval .... 0.10 second	S-T segment .... isoelectric

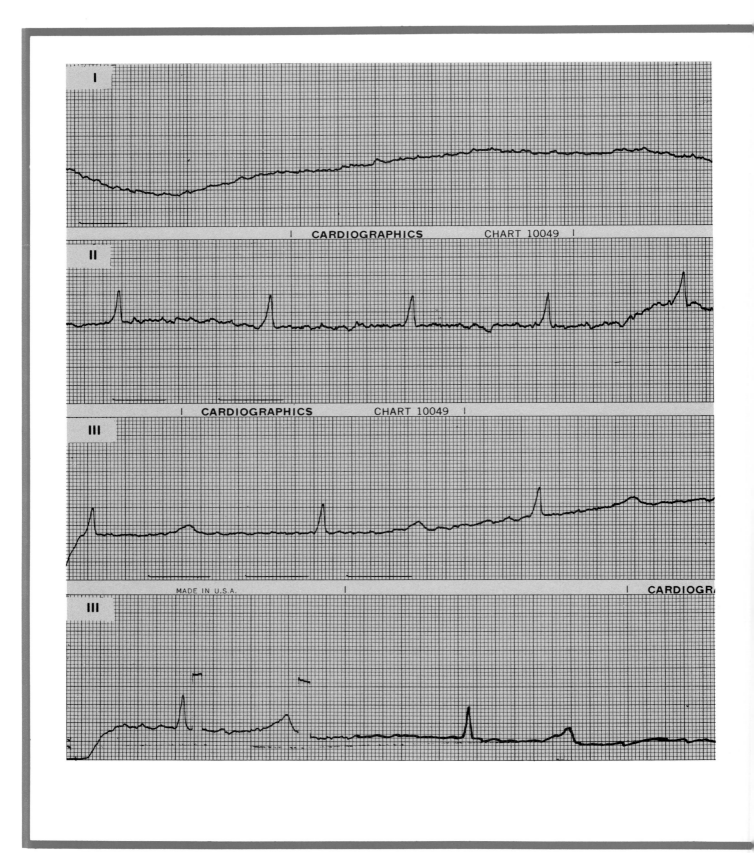

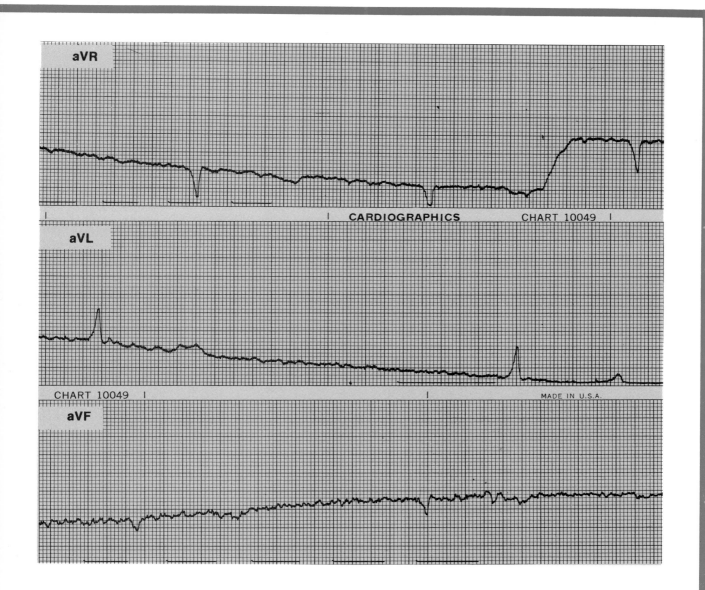

Figure 73
Clinically normal adult female red-eared slider (*Pseudemys scripta elegans*).

Ventricular rate .... approximately 40/minute

Q-R-S interval .... 0.12 second

R-wave amplitude .... 0.9 millivolt

Electrical axis .... approximately 40°

T-waves .... 0.24 second x 0.165 second

S-T segment .... isoelectric

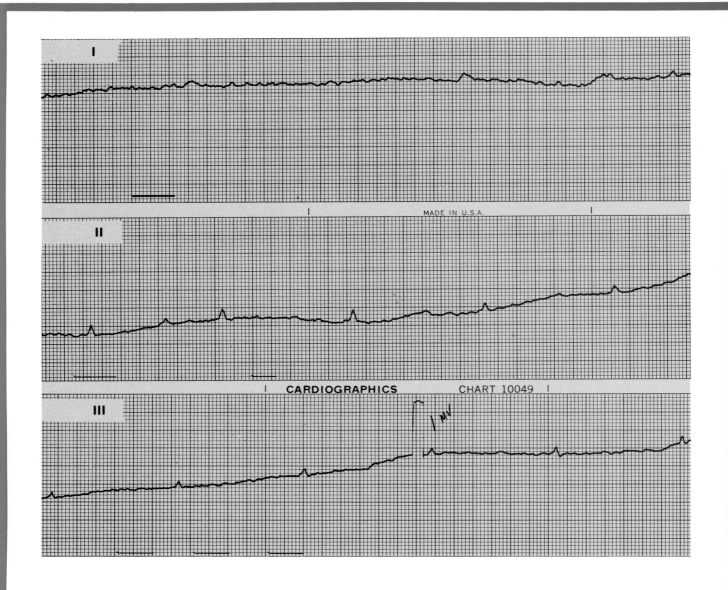

Figure 74
Adult female *Pseudemys scripta elegans* affected by chronic low dietary calcium. Note the diminished R-wave amplitude and decreased Q-R-S interval.

Ventricular rate . . . . 45/minute   R-wave amplitude . . . . 0.2 millivolt
Q-R-S interval . . . . 0.08 second   Electrical axis . . . . +60°

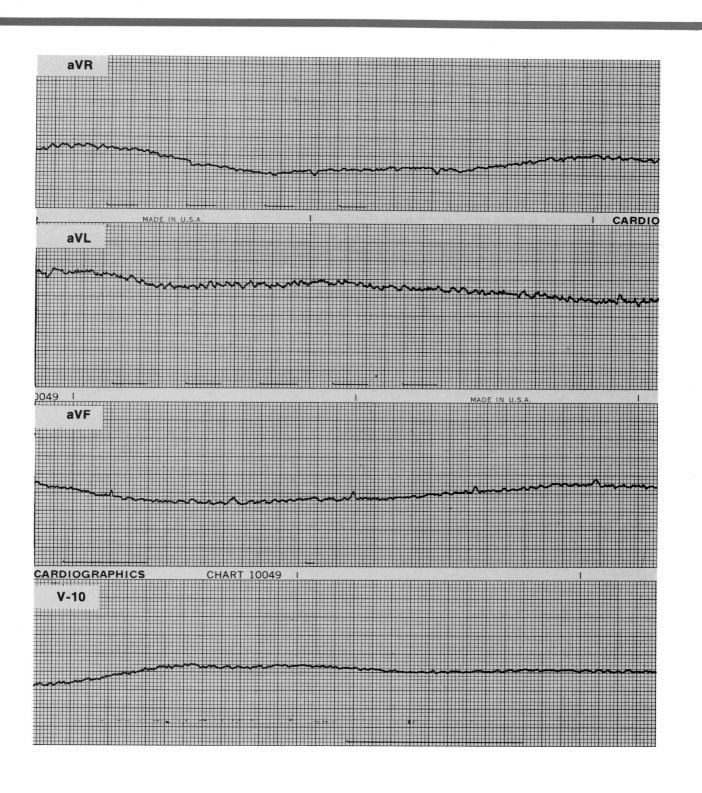

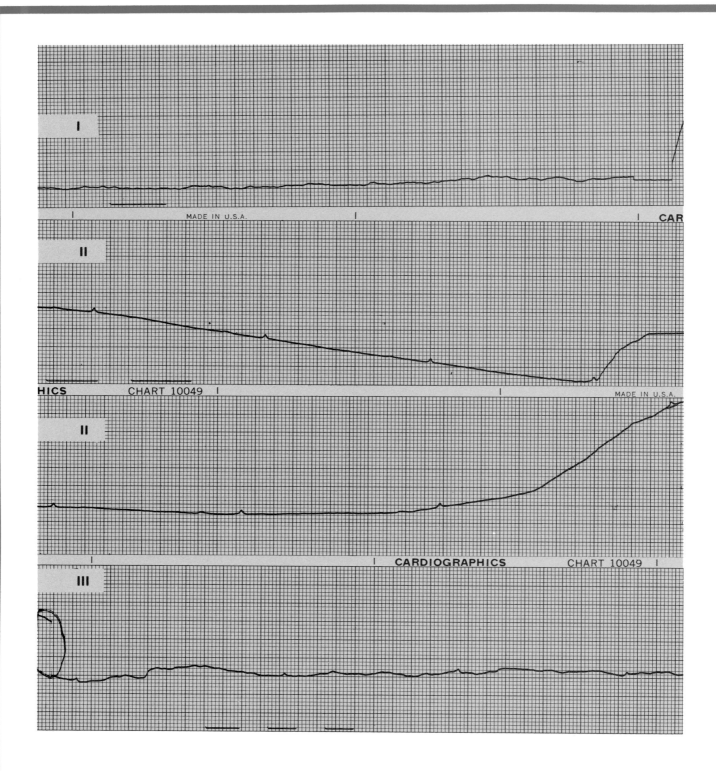

I

MADE IN U.S.A.

CAR

II

HICS   CHART 10049

II

MADE IN U.S.A.

CARDIOGRAPHICS   CHART 10049

III

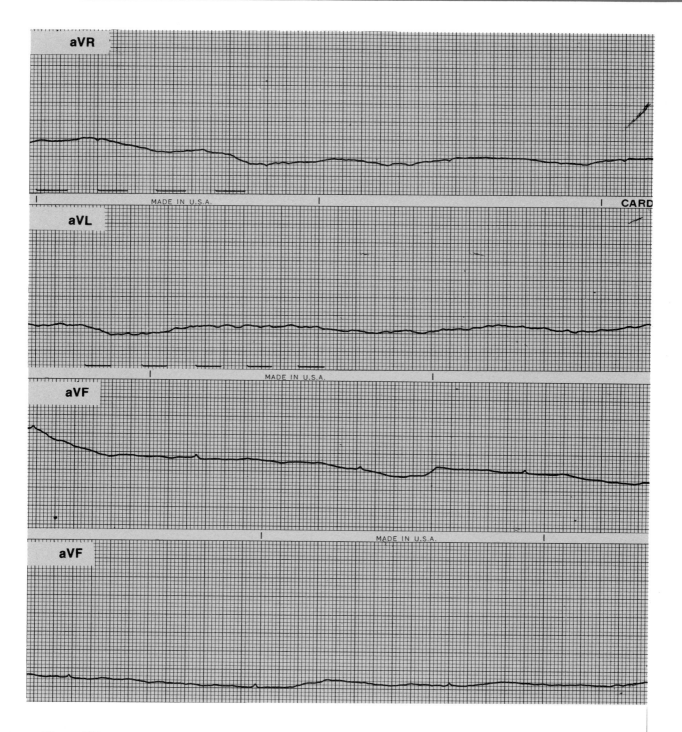

Figure 75

Young adult female western painted turtle (*Chrysemys marginata*) with chronic bronchopneumonia, atelectasis and unilateral (left) plural effusion. Note the greatly diminished R-wave amplitude.

Ventricular rate . . . . approximately 34/minute	R-wave amplitude . . . . 0.066 millivolt
P-R interval . . . . 0.44 second	Electrical axis . . . . approximately 60°
Q-R-S interval . . . . 0.06 second	S-T segment . . . . isoelectric

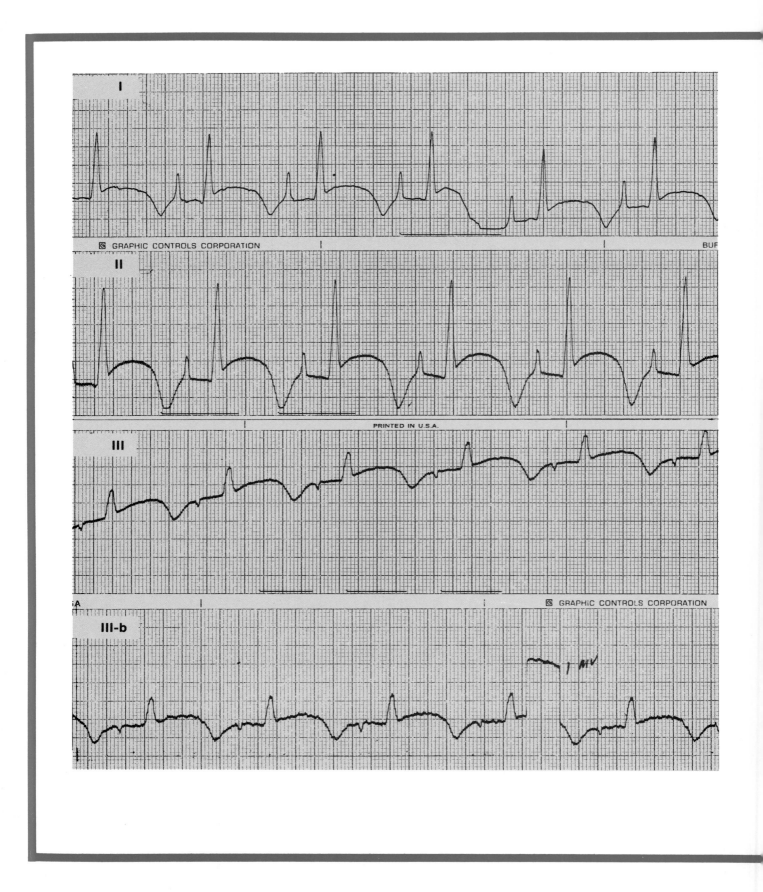

I

GRAPHIC CONTROLS CORPORATION   BUF

II

PRINTED IN U.S.A.

III

A   GRAPHIC CONTROLS CORPORATION

III-b

1 MV

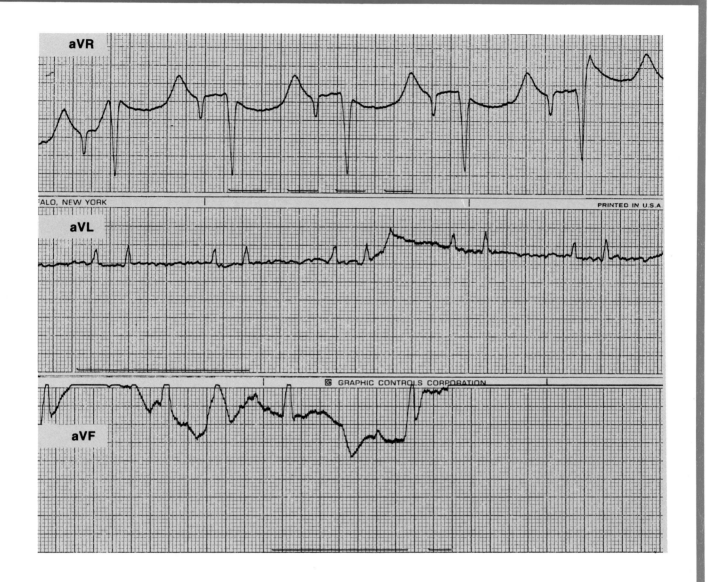

Figure 76
Adult indigo snake (*Drymarchon corais*); sex unknown.

Ventricular rate......... approximately 53/minute	R-wave amplitude .... approximately 2.5 millivolts
P-R interval .... 0.28 second	Electrical axis .... approximately 60°
Q-R-S interval .... 0.12 second	S-T segment .... +0.132 millivolt

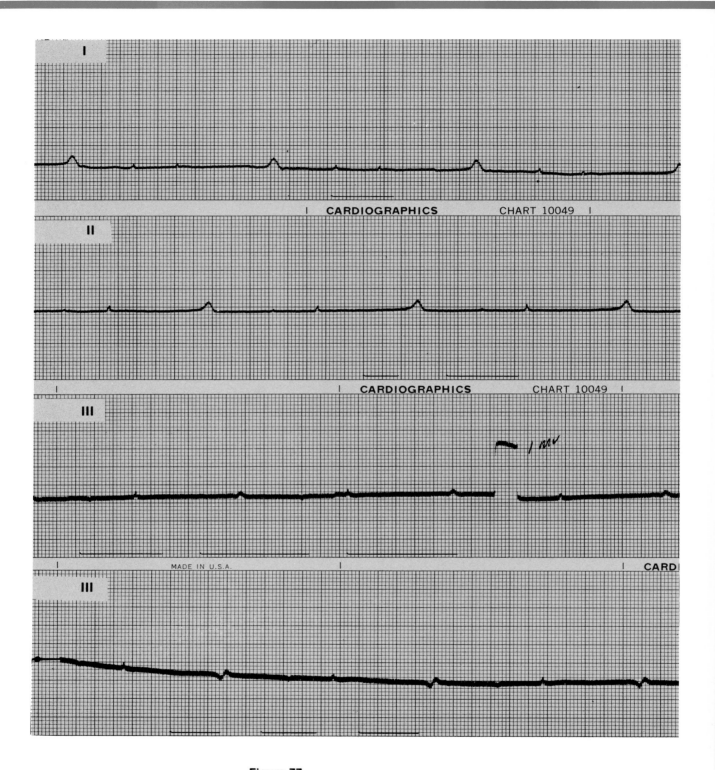

Figure 77
Immature female common iguana (*Iguana iguana*) affected by a chronic high-phosphorus/low-calcium dietary intake leading to fibrous osteodystrophy. Note the diminished R-wave amplitude and occasional ectopic abortive electrical activity interposed between Q-R-S complexes.

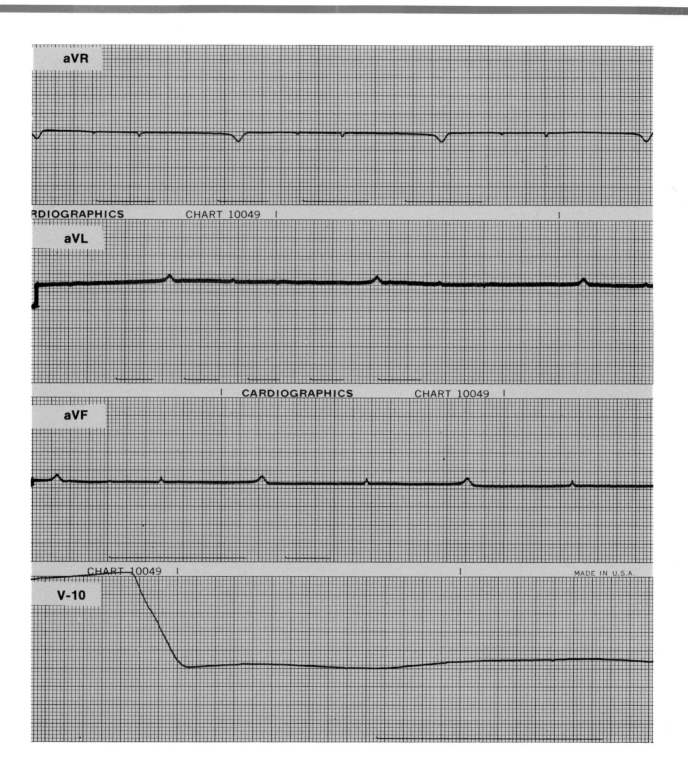

aVR	
aVL	
aVF	
V-10	

CARDIOGRAPHICS CHART 10049

CARDIOGRAPHICS CHART 10049

CHART 10049

MADE IN U.S.A.

Ventricular rate .... approximately 27/minute
P-R interval .... 0.96 second
Q-R-S interval .... 0.16 second
R-wave amplitude .... 0.132 millivolt

Electrical axis .... approximately 45°
S-T segment .... isoelectric
P-wave amplitude.................. 0.09 millivolt

PARENTERAL ANTIBIOTICS
Used in Captive Reptiles

Generic Name (Trade Name)	Source	Route	Frequency	Dosage	Remarks/ Precautions
Ampicillin trihydrate (Polyflex®)	Bristol	IM, SC	s.i.d. b.i.d.	3-6 mg/kg	
Benzathine penicillin with procaine penicillin (Flocillin®)	Bristol	IM	Varies with species and ambient temperature	10,000 units total penicillin activity/kg 24-72 hours	
Chloramphenicol (Chloromycetin® Succinate)	Parke-Davis	IV, IM	b.i.d. q.i.d.	10-15 mg/kg in divided doses	Should not be used in presence of impaired renal or hepatic function or dehydration
Gentamycin sulfate (Gentocin®)	Schering	IM, SC	b.i.d. 1st day; s.i.d. thereafter	4 mg/kg 1st day b.i.d.; s.i.d. next 2-6 days	Should not be used in presence of impaired renal or hepatic function or dehydration
Kanamycin sulfate (Kantrex®)	Bristol	IV, IM, IP; also as a wound-flushing agent	b.i.d. s.i.d.	10-15 mg/kg in divided doses	Should not be used in presence of impaired renal or hepatic function or dehydration
Lincomycin (Lincocin®)	Upjohn	IM	b.i.d. s.i.d.	6 mg/kg	Should not be used in presence of impaired renal or hepatic function or dehydration

Generic Name (Trade Name)	Source	Route	Frequency	Dosage	Remarks/ Precautions
Neomycin sulfate with polymyxin sulfate (Daribiotic®)	Beecham-Massengill	IM, IV; local wound-flushing agent	b.i.d. s.i.d.	10 mg/kg	Should not be used in presence of impaired renal or hepatic function or dehydration
Oxytetracycline hydrochloride; (Liquamycin® Injectable or Intramuscular)	Pfizer	IV, IM	s.i.d.	6-10 mg/kg	May produce some local inflammation at injection site
Potassium penicillin G.; Buffered U.S.P.	Squibb	IM, IP; local wound-flushing agent	Varies widely	20,000 - 80,000 units/kg	May cause cardiac arrest at high and rapid uptake dosages due to potassium ion
Streptomycin sulfate injectable U.S.P.	Squibb	IM	b.i.d.	10 mg/kg	Should not be used in presence of impaired renal or hepatic function or dehydration
Sulfadimethoxine (Symbio®)	Affiliated	IV, IM	s.i.d.	30 mg/kg 1st day; 15 mg/kg 2nd-4th day	Should not be used in presence of impaired renal or hepatic function or dehydration; hydration must be maintained

Generic Name (Trade Name)	Source	Route	Frequency	Dosage	Remarks/ Precautions
Acepromazine Maleate	Ayerst	IM	As required for tranquilization	0.125-0.5 mg/kg	Should not be used in animals recently exposed to organic phosphates
Aminophylline U.S.P.	G.D. Searle	IM; as suppository	As needed	2-4 mg/kg as required	
Ascorbic acid injection U.S.P.	Many	IM, SC	Varies widely; essentially nontoxic except for the sodium ion	Not established	
Atrophine sulfate injectable	Many	IM, IV, SC, oral	As needed	0.04 mg/kg	
Calcium gluconate injectable U.S.P.	Parke-Davis	IV, IM	As needed	500 mg/kg, in divided doses	May produce cardiac irregularities in rapid uptake time
Cyanocobalamin (Vit. B_{12})	Many	IM, SC	Not established	Not established; 10-2,000 units, depending on body weight	
Dexamethasone (Azium®)	Schering	IV, IM	As needed	0.0625-0.125 mg/kg	Should be used only when required
Furosemide (Lasix®)	National	IV, IM	As needed, s.i.d., b.i.d.	5 mg/kg	Hydration must be carefully observed
Furoxone® suspension	Eaton	Oral	s.i.d.	25-40 mg/kg	
Methischol	U.S. Vitamin and Pharmaceutical	Oral	As needed	A few drops to several ml/day, as required	Given to patients with hepatic lipodystrophy and infiltration

Generic Name (Trade Name)	Source	Route	Frequency	Dosage	Remarks/ Precautions
Prednisolone sodium succinate (Solu-Delta Cortef®)	Upjohn	IM, IV	As needed	Not established; 5-10 mg/kg as required	
Sodium iodide injectable	Burns-Biotec	IV	Not established	0.25-3 ml as required	
Stanozolol (Winstrol®)	Winthrop	IM	Varies with individual patient	Varies with individual patient	Should not be used in presence of impaired renal or hepatic function
Sulfamethazine solution	Merck	Oral	s.i.d.	0.5 gr./kg 1st day; 0.25 gr./kg 2nd, 3rd & 4th days	Should not be used in presence of impaired renal or hepatic function or dehydration
Sulfaquinoxyline solution	Merck	Oral	s.i.d.	0.04% in drinking water for 3 to 5 days	Should not be used in presence of impaired renal or hepatic function or dehydration
Vionate® powder or tablets	Squibb	Oral	With each feeding	Dosage varies with diet	
Vitamin A (Aquasol-A®)	U.S. Vitamin and Pharmaceutical	IM	Not established	1,000 U - 50,000 U	Overdosage may produce exostoses and hepatomegaly
Vitamin B complex	Parke-Davis	IM, IV, SC	Not established for prophylaxis	0.5 cc/kg	
Vitamin K (Synkamin®)	Parke-Davis	IM	Not established; as required	0.5 mg/kg (not established)	

TOPICAL OINTMENTS, SPRAYS AND SOLUTIONS Used in Captive Reptiles

Product	Manufacturer
Betadine® Solution	Purdue-Frederick
Dermafur® Ointment	Eaton
Dermalog® Ointment	Maurry
Elase® Ointment	Parke-Davis
Furacin® Dressing	Eaton
Furacin® Solution	Eaton
Kymar® Ointment	Armour
Panalog® Ointment	Squibb
Toptic® Ointment	Corvel

PARASITICIDES Used in Captive Reptiles

Generic Name (Trade Name)	Source	Route	Frequency	Dosage	Remarks/ Precautions
2,2-dichlorovinyl dimethyl phosphate (Vapona® Pest Strip)	Shell Chemical	Vapona-impregnated strips suspended above cages	Continuously	1 strip/ 1,000 cu. ft. room space	May be hazardous to humans having to breathe Vapona-laden air
Bunamidine HCl (Scolaban®)	Wm. Cooper & Nephews	Oral	Not more frequently than once every 2-3 weeks	25-50 mg/kg	Should not be used in animals with a known heart condition; effective against cestodes
Dichlorvos (Task®)	Shell Chemical	Oral	Daily for 2 doses	12.5 mg/kg	Should not be used in presence of impaired renal or hepatic function or dehydration
Emetine HCl Inj. U.S.P.	Eli Lilly & Co.	IM, SC	s.i.d. or b.i.d.	0.5 mg/kg daily for 10 days	Should not be used in debilitated patients or in known cases of renal disease; effective against some amoebae and trematodes
Niclosamide (Yomesan®)	Chemagro	Oral	Not more frequently than once/month	150 mg/kg	Effective against cestodes
Piperazine citrate	Many	Oral	As necessary; not to exceed once/2 weeks	40-60 mg/kg	
Tetrachlor-ethylene	Many	Oral	Not more frequently than once/month	0.2 ml/kg	Should not be used in presence of hepatic insufficiency
Thiabendazole (Thibenzole®)	Merck	Oral	As necessary	50 mg/kg	Use as a fluid drench

Bibliography

Altman, R., *et al*.: Turtle-Associated Salmonellosis. II. The Relationship of Pet Turtles to Salmonellosis in Children in New Jersey. *Am. J. Epidemiol. 95*:518-520; 1972.

Aronson, J.D.: Spontaneous Tuberculosis in Snakes. *J. Infect. Dis. 44*:215-223; 1929.

Ash, L.R.; Beaver, P.C.: A Restudy of *Ophidascaris labiatopapillosa* Occurring in the Stomach of North American Snakes. *J. Parasit. 48* (Suppl.): 41; 1962.

Ayala, S.C.: Lizard Malaria in California; Description of a Strain of *Plasmodium mexicanum,* and Biogeography of Lizard Malaria in Western North America. *J. Parasit. 56*:417-425; 1970.

Baker, E.F.; Anderson, H.W.; Allard, J.: Epidemiological Aspects of Turtle-Associated Salmonellosis. *Arch. Environ. Health 24*:1-9; 1972.

Ball, G.H.; Chao, J.; Telford, S.R., Jr.: The Life History of *Hepatozoon rarefaciens* (Sambon and Seligman, 1907) from *Drymarchon Corais* (*Colubridae*), and Its Experimental Transfer to *Constrictor constrictor* (*Boidae*). *J. Parasit. 53*:897-909; 1967.

Ball, G.H.; Chao, J.; Telford, S.R., Jr.: *Hepatozoon fusifex* sp. N., a Hemogregarine from Boa Constrictor Producing Marked Morphological Changes in Infected Erythrocytes. *J. Parasit. 55*:800-813; 1969.

Ball, G.H.; Oda, S.N.: Sexual Changes in the Life History of Hemogregarine *Hepatozoon rarefaciens* (Sambon and Seligman, 1907). *J. Protozool. 18*:698-700; 1971.

Bellairs, A. d'A.: Reptiles; in *The Universities Federation for Animal Welfare Handbook on Care and Management of Laboratory Animals.* E.S. Livingstone, London, England, 1967; pp. 830-852.

Bellairs, A. d'A: *The Life of Reptiles,* Vol. 1 and 2. Weidenfield and Nicolson, London, England, 1969.

Betz, T.W.: Surgical Anesthesia in Reptiles, with Special Reference to the Water Snake, *Natrix rhombifera. Copeia 2*:284-287; 1962.

Boam, G.W., *et al*.: Subcutaneous Abscesses in Iguanid Lizards. *JAVMA 157*:617-619; 1970.

Bonorris, J.S.; Ball, G.H.: *Schellackia occidentalis* n. sp., Blood-Inhabiting Coccidian Found in Lizards in Southern California. *J. Parasit. 2*:31-34; 1955.

Booden, T.; Chao, J.; Ball, G.H.: Transfer of a *Hepatozoon* sp. from Boa Constrictor to a Lizard, *Anolis carolinensis,* by Mosquito Vectors. *J. Parasit. 56*:832-833; 1970.

Bovee, E.C.; Telford, S.R., Jr.: *Eimeria sceloporis* and *Eimeria molochis* spp. n. from Lizards. *J. Parasitol. 51*:85-94; 1965.

Boycott, J.A.; Taylor, J.; Douglas, S.H.: Salmonella in Tortoises. *J. Path. & Bact. 65*:401-411; 1953.

Brisbin, I.L., Jr.: Reactions of the American Alligator to Several Immobilizing Drugs. *Copeia 1*:129-130; 1966.

Burke, T.J.; Wall, B.E.: Anesthetic Deaths in Cobras (*Naja naja* and *Ophiophagus hanna*) with Methoxyflurane. *JAVMA 157*:620-621; 1970.

Calderwood, H.W.: Anesthesia for Reptiles. *JAVMA 159*:1618-1625; 1971.

Camin, J.: Mite Transmission of a Haemorrhagic Septicaemia in Snakes. *J. Parasitol. 34*:345-354; 1948.

Camin, J.H., *et al*.: Control of the Snake Mite, *Ophionyssus natricis* (Gervais), in Captive Reptile Collections. *Zoologica 49*:65-79; 1964.

Chabaud, A.G.; Frank, W.: Nouvelle Filaire Parasite des Artères de Pythons: *Macdonaldius oscheri* n. sp. (Nematodes, Onchocercidae). *Ztschr. Parasiten 20*: 434-439; 1961.

Chao, J.; Ball, G.H.: Transfer of *Hepatozoon rarefaciens* (Sanbon and Seligmann, 1907) from the Indigo Snake to a Gopher Snake by a Mosquito Vector. *J. Parasitol. 55*:681-682; 1969.

Claussen, H.J.; Durand-Reynals, F.: Studies on the Experimental Infection of Some Reptiles, Amphibia, and Fish with *Serratia annollum. Am. J. Path. 13*:441-451; 1937.

Cowan, D.F.: Diseases of Captive Reptiles. *JAVMA 153*:848-859; 1968.

Doyle, R.E.; Moreland, A.F.: Diseases of Turtles. *Lab. Anim. Dig. 4*:3-6; 1968.

Fantham, H.B.; Porter, A.: The Endoparasites of Some North American Snakes and Their Effects on the Ophidia. *Proc. Zool. Soc. London 123*:867-898; 1953-1954.

Frank, W.: Die entwicklung von *MacDonaldius oscheri* Chabaud et Frank, 1961 (Filaroidea, Onchocercidae) in der Lederzelke *Ornithodoros talaje* [Guerin-Meneville (Ixodoidea, Argasidae)]. *Ztschr. Parasiten 24*:318-350; 1965b.

Frye, F.L.; Cucuel, J.P.E.; Uno, T.: A Gas Anesthesia Adapter for Small Animals. *JAVMA 151*:843-844; 1967.

Frye, F.L.: A Rapid Polymerizing Epoxy Resin for Repair of Shell Defects in Tortoises. *VM/SAC 68*:51-53; 1973.

Gandal, C.P.: A Practical Anesthetic Technique in Snakes, Utilizing Methoxyflurane. *Anim. Hosp. 4*:258-260; 1968.

Garnham, P.C.C.: *Malaria Parasites and Other Haemosporidia.* Blackwell, Oxford, England, 1966.

Hackenbrock, C.R.; Finster, M.: Fluothane: A Rapid and Safe Inhalation Anesthetic for Poisonous Snakes. *Copeia 2*:440-441; 1963.

Hansen, I.B.: The Breathing Mechanism of Turtles. *Science 94*:64; 1941.

Harrison, G.A.: Ayre's T-piece: A Review of Its Modifications. *Brit. J. Anaesth. 36*:115-120; 1964.

Hinsch, H.; Gandal, C.P.: The Effects of Etorphine (M.99), Oxymorphone Hydrochloride and Meperidine Hydrochloride in Reptiles. *Copeia* 2:404-405; 1969.

Hunt, T.J.: Notes on Diseases and Mortality in Testudines. *Herpetologica* 13:19-23; 1957.

Hunt, T.J.: Influence of Environment of Necrosis of Turtle Shells. *Herpetologica* 14:45-46; 1958.

Ippen, R.: Considerations on the Comparative Pathology of Bone Diseases in Reptiles. *Zentralbl. allg. Path.* 108:424-434; 1965.

Jackson, M.M.; Jackson, C.G., Jr.; Fulton, M.: Investigation of the Entire Bacteria of the Testudinea. I: Occurrence of the Genera *Arizona, Citrobacter, Edwardsiella* and *Salmonella. Bull. Wildlife Dis. Assn.* 5:328-329; 1969.

Jackson, C.G., Jr.; Jackson, M.M.: The Frequency of *Salmonella* and *Arizona* Microorganisms in Zoo Turtles. *J. Wildlife Dis.* 7:130-132; 1971.

Jackson, C.G., Jr.; Fulton, M.: A Turtle Colony Epizootic Apparently of Microbial Origin. *J. Wildlife Dis.* 6:466-468; 1970.

Jackson, C.G., Jr.; Fulton, M.; Jackson, M.M.: Cranial Asymmetry with Massive Infection in a Box Turtle. *J. Wildlife Dis.* 8:275-277; 1972.

Kaplan, H.M.: Septicemic Cutaneous Ulcerative Disease of Turtles. *Proc. Anim. Care Panel* 7:273-277; 1957.

Kaplan, H.M.: Treatment of Escherichiosis in Turtles, Frogs, and Rabbits. *Proc. Anim. Care Panel* 8:101-106; 1958.

Kaplan, H.M.: Anesthesia in Amphibians and Reptiles. *Fed. Proc.* 28:1541-1546; 1969.

Kaufmann, A.F.; Morrison, Z.L.: An Epidemiologic Study of Salmonellosis in Turtles. *Am. J. Epidemiol.* 84:364-370; 1966.

Kaufmann, A.F.; Feeley, J.C.; DeWitt, W.E.: *Salmonella* Excretion by Turtles. *Pub. Health Reports* 82:840-842; 1967.

Kraner, K.L.; Silverstein, A.M.; Parshall, C.J., Jr.: Surgical Anesthesia in Snakes. In *Experimental Animal Anesthesiology*, edited by D.C. Sawyer. USAF School of Aerospace Medicine, Brooks AFB, Texas, July 1965; pp. 374-378.

Lowenstein, M.S., *et al.*: Salmonellosis Associated with Turtles. *J. Infect. Dis.* 124:433; 1971.

Mackerras, M.J.: Haematozoa of Australian Reptiles. *Austral. J. Zool.* 9:61-122; 1961.

Marcus, L.C.: Diseases of Snakes and Turtles. In *Current Veterinary Therapy III*, edited by R.W. Kirk. W.B. Saunders Co., Philadelphia, Pa. 1968; pp. 435-442.

Marcus, L.C.: Infectious Diseases of Reptiles. *JAVMA* 159:1626-1631; 1971.

McCutcheon, F.H.: The Respiratory Mechanism in Turtles. *Physiol. Zool.* 16:255-269; 1943.

Mertens, R.: *The World of Amphibians and Reptiles.* McGraw-Hill Book Co., New York, N.Y., 1960.

Northway, R.B.: Electroanesthesia of Green Iguanas (*Iguana iguana*). *JAVMA* 155:1034; 1969.

Oda, S.N.; Chao, J.; Ball, G.H.: Additional Instances of Transfer of Reptile Hemogregarines to Foreign Hosts. *J. Parasit.* 57:1377-1378; 1971.

Page, L.A.: Experimental Ulcerative Stomatitis in King Snakes. *Cornell Vet.* 51:258-266; 1961.

Page, L.A.: Diseases and Infections of Snakes: A Review. *Bull. Wildlife Dis. Assn.* 2:111-126; 1966.

Pleuger, C.A.: Gastrotomy in a Crocodile: A Case Report. *JAVMA* 117:297-299; 1950.

Ratcliffe, H.L.; Geiman, Q.M.: Spontaneous and Experimental Amebic Infection in Reptiles. *Arch. Pathol.* 25:160-184; 1938.

Reichenbach-Klinke, H.; Elkan, B.: *The Principal Diseases of Lower Vertebrates.* Academic Press, Inc., New York, N.Y., 1965.

Rosenstein, B.J.; Russo, P.; Hinchliffe, M.C.: A Family Outbreak of Salmonellosis Traced to a Pet Turtle. *New Eng. J. Med.* 272:960-961; 1965.

Rothman, N.; Rothman, B.: Course and Care of Respiratory Infections in Snakes. *Philadelphia Herpet. Soc. Bull.* 8:19-23; 1960.

Schuchman, S.M.; Taylor, D.O.N.: Arteriosclerosis in an Iguana (*Iguana iguana*). *JAVMA* 157:614-616; 1970.

Shilkin, K.B.; Annear, D.I.; Rowett, L.R.: Infection Due to *Aeromonas hydrophila. Med. J. Austral.* 1:351-353; 1968.

Simmons, M.L.; Smith, L.H.: An Anesthetic Unit for Small Laboratory Animals. *J. Appl. Physiol.* 25:324-325; 1968.

Telford, S.R., Jr.: A Comparative Study of Endoparasitism Among Some Southern California Lizard Populations. *Am. Midl. Nat.* 83:516-554; 1970.

Telford, S.R., Jr.: Parasitic Diseases of Reptiles. *JAVMA* 159:1644-1652; 1971.

Wallach, J.D.: Medical Care of Reptiles. *JAVMA* 155:1017-1032; 1969.

Wallach, J.D.; Hoessle, C.: M.99 as an Immobilizing Agent in Poikilothermes. *VM/SAC* 65:163-167; 1970.

Wenyon, C.M.: *Protozoology. A Manual for Medical Veterinarians and Zoologists, Vol. II.* Wood & Co., New York, N.Y., 1926; pp. 1109-1110.

Zeman, W.V.; Falco, F.G.; Falco, J.J.: Repair of the Carapace of a Box Turtle Using a Polyester Resin. *Lab. Anim. Care.* 17:424-425; 1967.

SURGERY & PATHOLOGY

Anesthesia

Reptiles *can* Perceive Pain!

1. Local Anesthesia

Field or line blocks with 2% lidocaine are effective for fairly minor procedures in the smaller snakes, lizards and crocodilia—if adequate restraint is provided.

Digital amputations have been accomplished in a number of alligators at Steinhart Aquarium using only lidocaine for anesthesia. On one occasion, I amputated the left rear leg of an American alligator at midfemur using only lidocaine at progressively deeper infiltration levels (*Figure 78*). The anesthetic worked well, but maintaining total restraint of the 360-lb. animal was cumbersome. If the use of fluothane (Halothane®—Ayerst) is anticipated, lidocaine with epinephrine should not be used, as cardiac irregularities may be induced.

2. General Anesthesia

Many anesthetic agents, both injectable and gaseous, have been tried and found safe and effective. Those discussed here are those which have given consistently good results. The objective should always be patient safety, rapid induction, and reasonably rapid recovery after withdrawal of the agent. Ketamine hydrochloride, at a dosage of 20-40 mg./kg. injected intramuscularly, is useful in some of the smaller captive reptiles. Induction time, duration of anesthesia, and recovery time are not entirely predictable, but generally it will allow for about 30 to 60 minutes of chemical restraint at room temperature.

M.99 (Etorphine®—American Cyanamid) has been my favorite anesthetic agent for use in alligators and caimans. Induction requires about 15 to 30 minutes when M.99 is administered intramuscularly, less when it is injected intraperitoneally. The recommended dosage is 0.05 to 2.0 mg. for small alligators, with up to 36 mg. being given to a large female alligator weighing 337 pounds. Both dosage and induction time can be reduced significantly by utilizing intraperitoneal injection. Recovery usually occurs about one hour after the onset of maximum effect. If a long procedure is anticipated, supplemental gas anesthesia, delivered via a closed system with positive-pressure assistance, is advantageous and safe. I modified a Heidbrink Kinet-O-Meter® and added a Bird Mark 7® assist respirator so that safe ventilation is assured. Induction is accomplished with 3% to 4% halothane.

A 3:1 nitrous oxide-oxygen mixture is also practical and safe when delivered by the Heidbrink-Bird Mark 7 combination. As soon as possible, the nitrous oxide is discontinued and the halothane is decreased to 1.5% to 2.0%.

A gas anesthesia adapter is useful for induction. A chamber may also be used for smaller patients. Endotracheal intubation should be performed as soon as possible after induction.

Presurgical Preparation of Reptilian Patients

The skin of many reptiles is heavily contaminated with a plethora of organisms because of their aquatic habits and/or scaliness. The most acceptable method of preparing the skin or shell consists of sufficiently repeated scrubs with a detergent or a surgical soap containing iodine, followed by application of an aqueous or alcoholic mixture containing a surgical antiseptic. I prefer povidone-iodine surgical scrubs followed by a swabbing with povidone-iodine solution.

Draping with towels and a fenestrated surgical drape should be routine whenever possible. Surgical instruments, gauze sponges, and sutures should be sterile. The operative technique is the same as for mammalian patients.

There is no mitigating excuse for employing sloppy, nonsterile surgical technique with reptiles. Successful surgical results will reward the inventive and meticulous surgeon.

Amputations

Amputations of the tail and/or a single limb often must be performed as a result of advanced wound infection which has led to gangrenous involvement of distal segments (*Figures 79a & 79b, 80a*).

If a limb must be sacrificed to save a patient's life, I prefer to make the section as high as possible. In the forelimb, the scapulo-humeral articulation is the preferred site; if the hindlimb is to be removed, then the upper one-third of the femur, or the coxofemoral joint, is the most favorable location. These techniques insure maximum postoperative ambulatory comfort and freedom from undesirable sequellae.

Careful attention must be paid to insure that adequate normal skin is available for final closure. Two curvilinear incisions, which create flaps, are made at the beginning of surgery. These two incisions are joined at each end. If possible, transection is not done through the belly of the muscles; rather, the sections are made through the relatively avascular tendinous portions at the distal ends of the muscles. Major vascular structures are ligated in routine fashion to prevent major blood loss and aid in primary healing. Appropriate instrumentation is used for either disarticulating the limb or for transecting the major long bone.

After satisfactory hemostasis has been achieved, the two curved skin flaps are closed starting in the *center* and working on alternate sides of the center toward the anterior and posterior ends of the flaps. This method creates a pucker-free skin closure. Nonabsorbable sutures are placed as close together as necessary. In most cases, the sutures are removed in three to four weeks. In semi-aquatic species, such as the crocodilia, the sutures are left in place for a longer time. Dressings are usually contraindicated.

When a segment of a tail must be removed, the site of transection is proximal to the line of demarcation between healthy and diseased tissue. The coccygeal elements are disarticulated proximal to the transection of soft tissue, and the soft tissues are then approximated so that they cover the distal bony element. The curvilinear skin flaps are closed as for amputation of a limb. Hemorrhage is rarely a problem in tail amputations in lizards since many lizards can shed their tails as a defense maneuver. The coccygeal vessels will rarely bleed for more than a moment or two. Hemostasis is accomplished via automatic constriction of these vessels.

When snake skin is being sutured, an attempt should be made to create a slight everting pattern. There is a natural tendency for the skin of serpents to curl slightly inward when incised. The sutures should be removed when the incision has healed, as their presence may impede the normal shedding of skin in the future.

Miscellaneous Procedures

Overgrowth of the horny maxillary and mandibular beaks of turtles and tortoises is a frequently-encountered management problem (*Figures 80c-80e*). Treatment consists of trimming these overgrowths with appropriate scissors or shears.

Split or segmental defects involving the horny beak are easily repaired by using epoxy resin. This material is virtually biologically inert, wears very well in daily use, and is cosmetically acceptable (*Figure 53*).

Infrequently, large defects in the maxilla arise from chronic abscessation (*Figure 46e*). These defects produce communications between the oral cavity and the outside. Treatment consists of debridement and prosthetic replacement with epoxy resin.

The claws of chelonians and saurians occasionally will become overgrown (*Figure 80c*). Trimming with nail clippers is effective and rarely must be performed more than once yearly.

Paraphimosis of the penis and prolapse of the cloaca sometimes occur in reptiles (*Figures 80f & 80g*). If the prolapsed tissue appears to be viable, routine cleansing of the outer, exposed surface with Betadine® solution, followed by the application of crystal glycerine or 50% dextrose solution, will allow for reasonably simple replacement. Ophthalmic antibiotic ointment also may be used as a lubricant, but prolapses recur more often after its use than after the use of a nonlipid such as glycerine.

Purse-string sutures may be placed in the circumcloacal tissues to prevent prolapses.

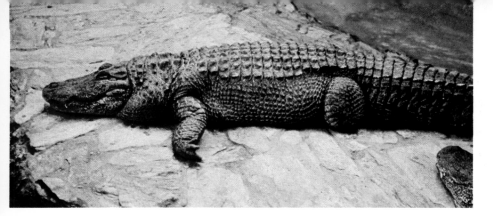

Figure 78—Midfemoral amputation in a mature American alligator.

Figures 79a & 79b—Scapulohumeral amputation in a chuckwalla: a) massive bacterial infection with gangrene in the right foreleg; b) post-surgical appearance.

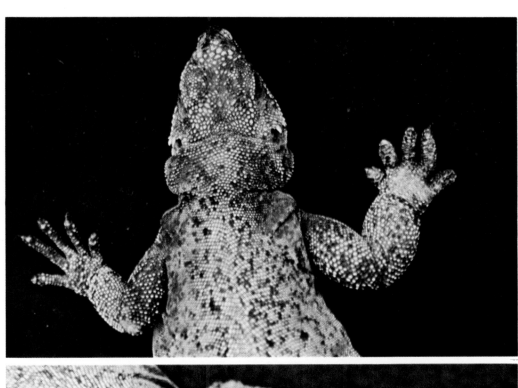

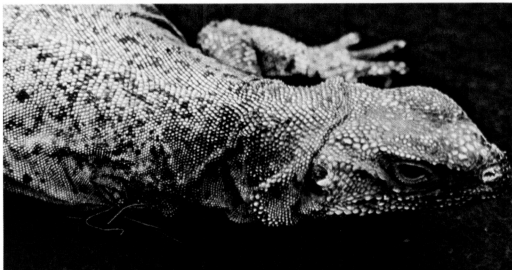

The sutures are removed one week later.

If the prolapsed tissue is obviously necrotic, amputation to the beginning of the healthy tissue is the treatment of choice. Suturing usually is not necessary. Local and parenteral antibiotic therapy should be employed until healing is complete.

Inclusion cysts involving the tail of captive iguanid lizards are seen frequently. The etiology is not known, but evidence suggests that poor husbandry practices, such as chronic dampness, poor cage hygiene, and failure to encourage or aid in the complete shedding of skin, may be predisposing causes. Parasitic bites also have been suggested, but not proven,

as etiologic factors. These lesions appear as solitary or multiple solid nodules involving the tail tissues from skin to deeper muscular and fascial structures. Treatment consists of either local excision, if possible, or caudectomy to a point of normal healthy tissue.

Occasionally, a venomous snake is presented for excision of the venom glands and the associated ducts. I have refused to perform such surgery for several reasons. The nature of the surgery must be considered to be not in the best interest of the patient and/or the surgeon. The venom glands are modified salivary glands. They are an integral portion of the food-gathering function of snakes, help-

Miscellaneous Conditions (*Figures 80a-80l*)

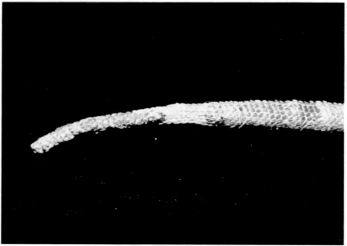

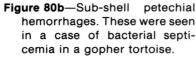

Figure 80a—Dry gangrene of the tail of lizards is a relatively common finding. The cause is not always apparent, but a history of trauma is common.

Figure 80b—Sub-shell petechial hemorrhages. These were seen in a case of bacterial septicemia in a gopher tortoise.

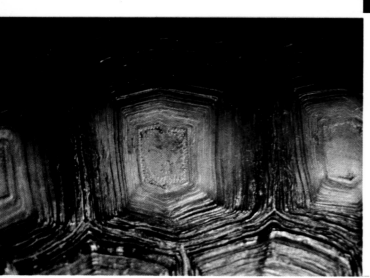

ing in the capture and immobilization of prey, and in many cases, aiding in digestion.

The medico-legal aspects of such surgery must be considered. If a person should be envenomated by a snake on which amputation of the venom glands has been performed (or a snake which is represented as being the same snake), the clinician involved must bear the burden of proof that he was in no way liable for injury through negligence on his part. Remaining glandular tissue or accessory glandular tissue could prove to be disastrous. Finally, willful mutilation of any species

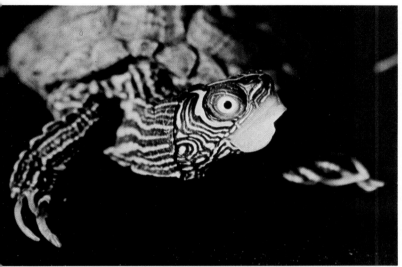

Figures 80c to 80e
Overgrowth of the horny mouth
parts and claws.

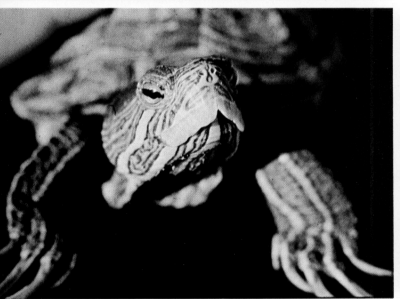

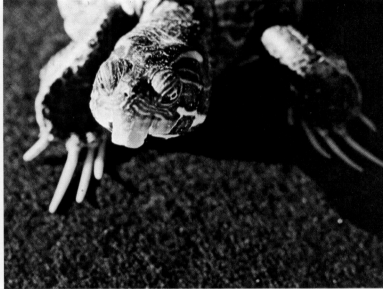

should be condemned.

The simple extraction of the fangs of venomous snakes and lizards also is discouraged on the same grounds. These teeth are deciduous and eventually will be replaced. In the interim, the smaller, non-fang teeth can puncture skin sufficiently to permit percutaneous envenomation to occur by way of wound contamination.

Following surgery, the patient must be observed during the immediate anesthetic recovery period. An elevated ambient temperature may be desirable in many cases, but should not be increased until voluntary respiration has been established. Respiratory stimulation with small amounts of pentylenetetrazol may be helpful.

After the patient has returned to consciousness, recovery with a minimum of handling or disturbance is desirable. It is helpful to provide a dark hiding place in the cage for a few days. Return to feeding may be either immediate or prolonged. If circumstances warrant it, hand-feeding may be advisable.

Observation for wound infection, drainage or abnormal swelling is routine.

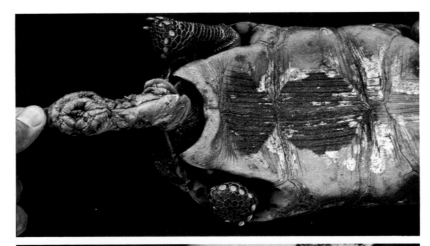

Figure 80f
Paraphimosis in a male tortoise.

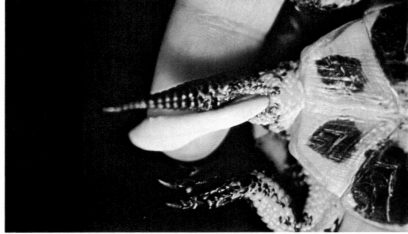

Figure 80g
Paraphimosis in a male turtle.

Figure 80h
Massive hydropic degeneration
of the liver; etiology unknown.

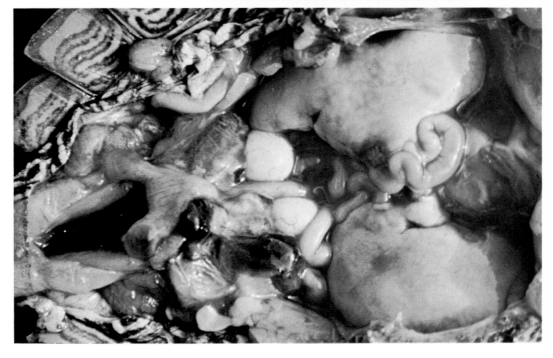

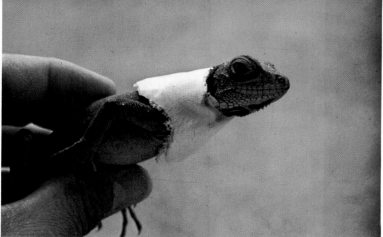

Figure 80i—Method of splinting the forelimb in a lizard or crocodilian for repair of a simple fracture. The affected leg is immobilized in a natural position next to the thorax.

Figure 80j—A radiograph showing gastroliths in a caiman. This condition is not pathologic.

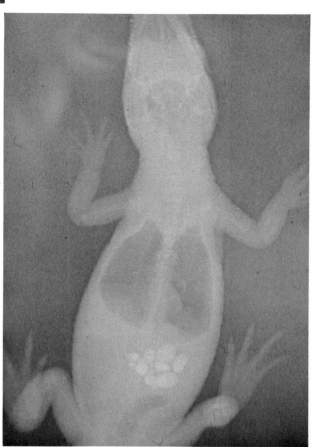

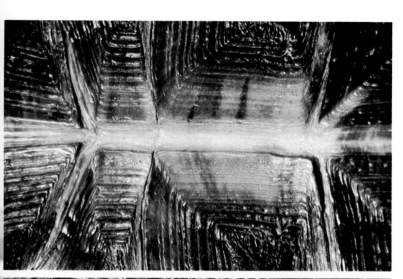

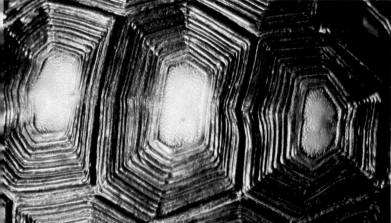

Figures 80k & 80l—Normal growth sites in the shell of a tortoise. Figure k: the plastron; note the white-growth interface. Figure l: the carapace. Growth occurs between the outermost rings in each plate.

Surgery

A. Chelonians

For incisions through the shell of chelonians, we use a hand-held rotary power saw. The blade is cooled by the constant application of a chilled irrigating solution consisting of lactated Ringer's solution to which Daribiotic® (Beecham-Massengill) has been added at a dilution of 5 ml. Daribiotic® to 1 liter of Ringer's solution.

Once the shell has been incised, the soft tissues are operated on as in the homothermic species. Catgut and polyglycolic suture materials are well tolerated.

Shell closure is accomplished routinely, as already mentioned, with fiberglass fabric impregnated with Devco® "5-Minute" epoxy resin (*Figures 81a-81j*).

After primary healing of shell defects has occurred, the epoxy resin-fiberglass patches should be either: 1) removed entirely; 2) relieved with a rotary burr or routed down to healthy shell to allow continuation of normal growth along growth zones at the interfaces of the rings. To ascertain that sufficient healing has progressed, postoperative radiographs should be made before the epoxy is removed.

B. Crocodilia

In crocodilia, celiotomies may be necessary for exploratory reasons, gastrotomies, etc. I have used a "window-flap" method of incision to afford greater exposure. This is necessary because of the distal and ventral excursion of the ribs in these species. Two transverse paracostal incisions are made and joined at the midline with a single ventral midline incision.

Closure is routine. Either very heavy Vetafil®(Dr. S. Jackson) or stainless monofilament wire is used. Wire is preferable if the patient is large and the surface of the enclosure is very abrasive. The sutures are placed between the dermal plates with a heavy cutting-edge needle. The incision may be sealed additionally with Eastman 910 Medical Monomer Adhesive® (Eastman-Kodak). Where applicable, flank incisions may also be employed in the saurian species.

The patient should not be put into water for several days. Water may be given orally via a garden hose.

C. Lizards

In lizards with dry gangrenous lesions involving portions of the tail and toes, amputations can be performed much the same as in the dog and cat. The coccygeal vertebrae or digits are trimmed back more proximally than the overlying soft tissues so that a soft, padded terminus is produced.

Skin closure is accomplished with nonabsorbable sutures of appropriate size for the patient. Tycon®(Davis & Geck) cardiovascular suture material, a silicone-treated polyester furnished with a swaged-on atraumatic needle, is highly recommended (*Figures 82a-82f*).

Almost all surgical procedures are possible and practical in reptiles. The only limiting factors are the economic practicality and the interest and zeal of the clinician.

Euthanasia

There are occasions when a captive reptile must be sacrificed. Safety for the operator, humane dispatch of the animal, and salvage of the specimen for pathologic examination or preservation are all valid considerations.

Venomous species can be euthanatized by saturation of their airspace with chloroform, ether, methoxyflurane, halothane or other volatile gases. Practicality, freedom from fire hazard, and low cost can be served with the use of chloroform. The length of time required to induce loss of consciousness varies with the species, ambient temperature, partial pressure of the anesthetic agent, etc., but usually is brief.

A swift and efficient method for rendering a reptile insensitive is the injection of a small amount of alcohol through the foramen magnum. Intraperitoneal injection of a concentrated barbiturate solution is also satisfactory.

With most methods, the reptilian heart continues to beat for a long time after the animal loses consciousness. This factor makes circulating blood readily available for study.

Necropsy Technique

Mortui vivos docent!

Surely not all patients will benefit from the veterinarian's ministrations. In many cases, besides affording the clinician the opportunity to make a definitive diagnosis (albeit postmortem), a thorough exploration of the reptile cadaver can lead to familiarity with the anatomy of each major reptilian group for future reference when dealing with live patients. Whenever possible, a necropsy should be performed; medicine, surgery, radiology and pathology all benefit.

Whenever possible, whole blood should be obtained and placed in collection tubes containing EDTA.

A. Chelonians

The highly specialized chelonians provide a plethora of individualized adaptations to the confinement created by the unyielding shell. Even the extremely pliant soft-shelled turtles *Trionyx* show marked individual variation between species, brought about by their particular dorsoventral flattening. The Pakistani Urdu word for these turtles is "chapati," a tortilla-like unleavened bread. The description is apt.

In the aquatic species, the placement of the lungs over most of the dorsal and dorsolateral expanse of the carapace—extending from the cranial to the most caudal curvature of the shell—affords a large area for exchange of respiratory gases, as well as a very useful hydrostatic organ. A state of positive, neutral

Cystotomy in a Desert Tortoise (*Figures 81a-81j*)

Figures 81a & 81b—Preoperative radiographs. Note the large, laminated calculus.

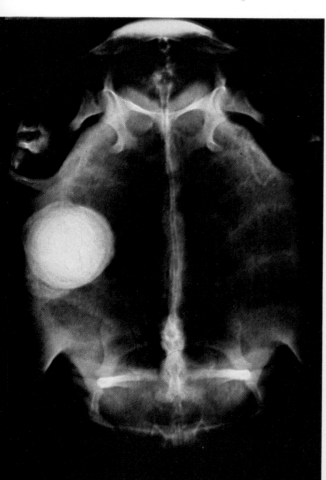
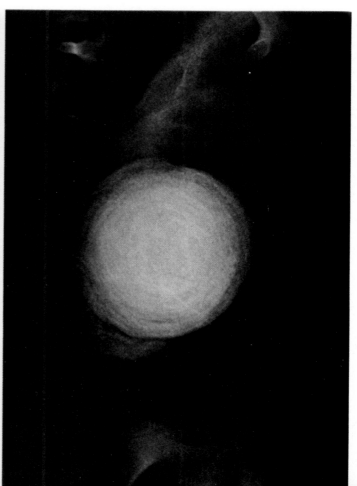

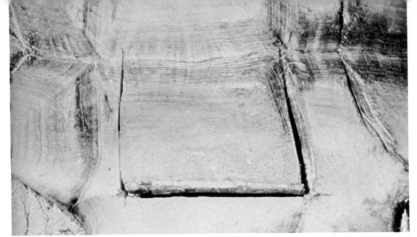

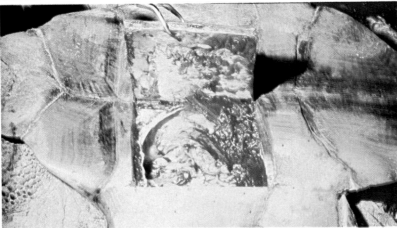

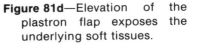

Figure 81c—After thorough preoperative preparation, an orthopedic saw was used to cut a hole through the plastron. (Surgical drapes were removed for the purpose of photography only.)

Figure 81d—Elevation of the plastron flap exposes the underlying soft tissues.

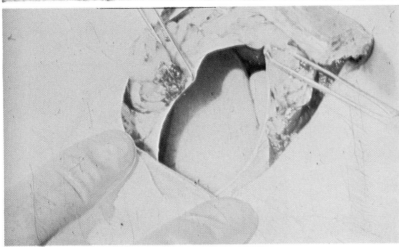

Figure 81e—Peritoneal incision. The large bowel is immediately below the peritoneum.

Figure 81f—The cystic calculus after removal from the urinary bladder.

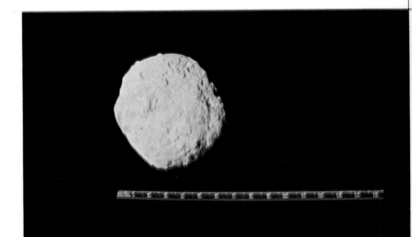

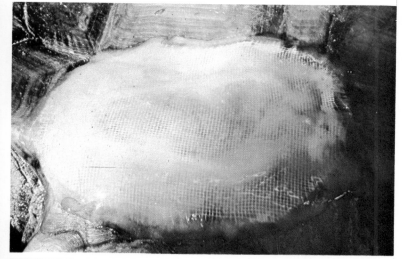

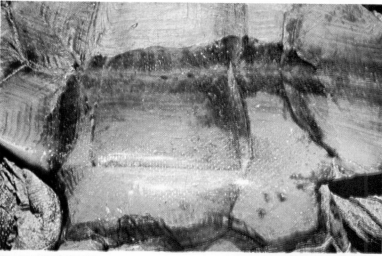

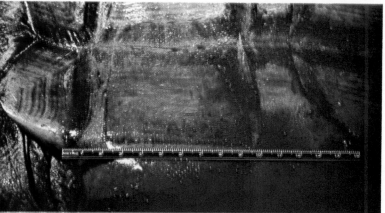

Figures 81g to 81i—Steps in shell repair.

Figure g: application of epoxy-impregnated fiberglass strips;

Figure h: additional epoxy resin is applied to the patch;

Figure i: the completed repair.

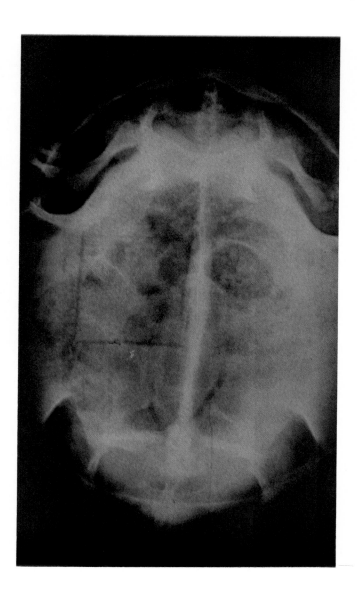

Figure 81j—A radiograph made one year postoperatively. The shell incision has been almost completely replaced by new bone.

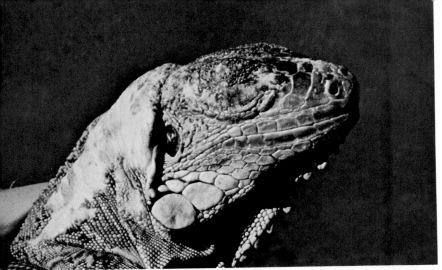

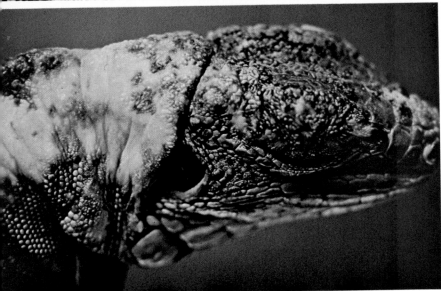

Blepharoplasty in an Iguana Severely Burned by an Overhead Heat Lamp

(Figures 82a-82f)

Figures 82a & 82b—Preoperative appearance. Note the massive scarring on the right side of the head and neck. Structures of the right eyelid are missing.

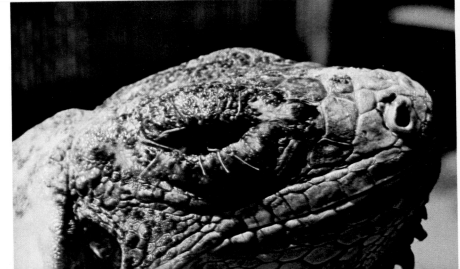

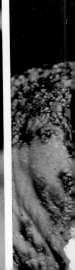

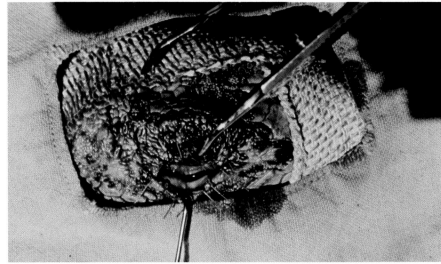

Figure 82c
Dissection between eyelid tissues to delineate the mucocutaneous margins.

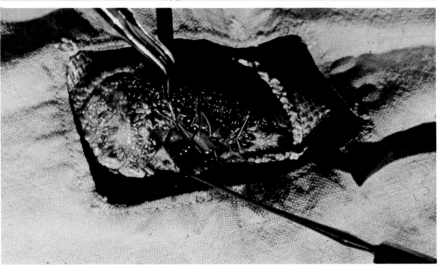

Figure 82d
New lid margins were created by suturing upper and lower mucous and cutaneous margins to their respective partners.

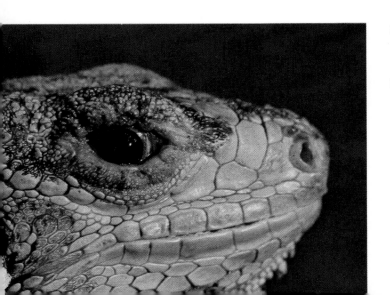

Figure 82e—The completed blepharoplasty immediately after surgery.

Figure 82f—The postoperative appearance eight and one-half weeks after surgery.

or negative buoyancy can be achieved by the relative expansion or contraction of the pulmonary bed.

In chelonians, a Stryker reciprocating cast-cutting or orthopedic saw can be used to divide the carapace from the plastron. A hand-saw can also be used. Using a flexible boning knife, the underlying musculature is severed; this allows the plastron to be lifted free. The beast is thus revealed "on the half shell," so to speak.

B. Crocodilia and Saurians

Crocodilia and saurians are examined in the routine fashion, utilizing the previously described ventral midline incision joining two transverse paracostal incisions. (*See Crocodilia, page 120.*)

C. Serpents

Snake cadavers can usually be examined thoroughly via a ventral midline incision extending from the intramandibular fossa to just caudal to the cloacal vent.

D. Organs of Reptilian Species

1. Alimentary Tract

a. Oral Cavity and Pharynx

A search should be made for evidence of stomatitis, dental and gingival infection, neoplasia, deformities, foreign bodies and parasites.

b. Esophagus and Stomach

The esophagus is characterized by well-developed folds running longitudinally to the stomach, which is simple and S-shaped in all reptilians but the snakes. The stomach of the snake is fusiform. Rugae are poorly developed. Ulcers are a common finding in crocodilia and snakes. Gastroliths are commonly seen in the crocodilia and are not pathologic (*Figure 80j*). Parasites are a frequent finding.

c. Liver

The large bilobed liver is seen in all the reptilians but snakes, in which the liver is fusiform. Usually occupying a site between the heart, anteriorally, and the stomach, posteriorally, the liver usually is dark-red in color, but may be yellowish-brown in cases of steatitis and hepatic lipodystrophy.

d. Gallbladder

The gallbladder is present in all reptiles. The common bile duct enters the duodenum.

e. Pancreas

The pancreas is pink in color, and occupies a position alongside the duodenum.

f. Small Intestine

The small intestine terminates at the ileocolic juncture.

g. Large Intestine

The large bowel enters the proctodeum, which in turn empties into the cloaca. Parasites may be found throughout the hollow viscera, as well as free within the coelom.

2. Respiratory System

a. Nasal Cavity

The nasal cavity should be examined via a transverse section across the maxilla. Upper respiratory parasites are a common finding.

b. Glottis

A well-developed glottis is prominent in most reptiles. In crocodilia, a muscular and cartilaginous valve seals both the respiratory and alimentary system when the mouth is opened and the tongue is depressed. This is an aquatic adaptation.

c. Trachea

As in other species, the trachea of the reptile continues to the bronchi.

d. Lungs

The lungs arise from the primary bronchi which may branch to secondary bronchi from a mesobronchus. In snakes, the left lung may be poorly developed. The lungs of lizards and crocodilia are more highly developed. In snakes and chelonians, the dorsal surface of the lungs may be attached to the ribs, and the lateral surface may be attached to the carapace musculature. Parasites, mucopus, foreign bodies and pigment may be found throughout the respiratory tract.

3. Cardiovascular System

Chelonians, lizards and snakes possess a three-chambered heart with two atria and a single well-developed ventricle. In the chelonians, a large sinus venosus is present. Crocodilia have a primitive four-chambered heart with an incomplete ventricular septum separating the two ventricles.

Blood leaving the heart exits via three main trunks, each of which has a single row of semilunar valves at its base. One trunk is the pulmonary aorta which divides into two pulmonary arteries going to the lungs. The pulmonary aorta leaves the right side of the ventricle. The two remaining trunks are called the left and right aortae, respectively. The left aorta leads from the right side of the ventricle, and the right aorta leads from the left side.

The right aortic arch, carrying oxygenated blood from the left ventricle, gives off a large brachiocephalic artery which distributes blood to the anterior part of the body.

At the base of the brachiocephalic trunk arise small coronary arteries which pass to the myocardium.

A coronary sinus returns blood to the right atrium.

Some mixing of arterial and venous blood occurs in all reptiles.

4. Endocrine System

a. Hypophysis

The hypophysis is located on the cranial floor near the origin of the optic nerve.

b. Thyroid Gland

The thyroid gland is found just cranial to the heart near the tracheal bifurcation. It is deep-pink to dark-red in color.

c. Adrenal Glands

The paired adrenal glands are found in the mesorchium, just caudomedial to the gonads.

5. Genitourinary System

a. Kidneys

Paired, lobulated kidneys are found in all reptiles. Ureters empty into a urinary bladder or directly into the urodeum of the cloaca. In snakes, the right kidney is cranial to the left kidney.

b. Testes or Ovaries

The testes or ovaries are located medial to the kidneys on either side of the caudal vena cava. In some lizards, the testes or ovaries may be situated quite anterior to the kidneys. The gonads are white-to-yellow in color and usually are attached to the kidney by the mesorchium.

In most snakes, the testes are located posterior to the cloacal vent. They may be bifid for approximately one-half their length, with the Y-shaped end lying posteriorly. In most snakes, a dark-colored scent gland is associated with each testicle and hemipenis. The color of the testicle is usually grayish-pink.

In adult females, developing yellowish egg follicles may be seen. The oviducts in the female, and the vas deferens in the male, exit directly into the caudal cloaca and hemipenes, respectively. Female crocodilia possess a small, pigmented clitoris-like papilla which has a tiny orifice on either side at its base.

6. Central Nervous System

The relatively small brain is most easily removed after the cranium has been cut in a saggital plane.

7. Hemopoietic Organs

a. Spleen

The spleen is usually a small, spherical, red organ lying between the pancreas and gallbladder. It is attached to the dorsal mesentery.

b. Bone Marrow

Bone marrow is located in the long bones and spinal vertebral bodies. It is best studied by examining stained decalcified tissue sections.

E. Neoplasia

While there are few reports of histopathologically-confirmed neoplasms in reptiles, both benign and malignant tumors do occur in all members of the order. One of the most common tumors seen in captive alligators, caimans, and alligator snapping turtles is the foot-pad fibroma. Whether this tumor is a true neoplasm or an environmentally-induced lesion is a moot point. These lesions are usually somewhat ulcerated and tend to bleed when only slightly abraded. Removal is done in a routine manner.

We recently diagnosed myeloproliferative disease with frank leukemia in a small turtle (*Figures 83a-83l*), and lymphocytic leukemia

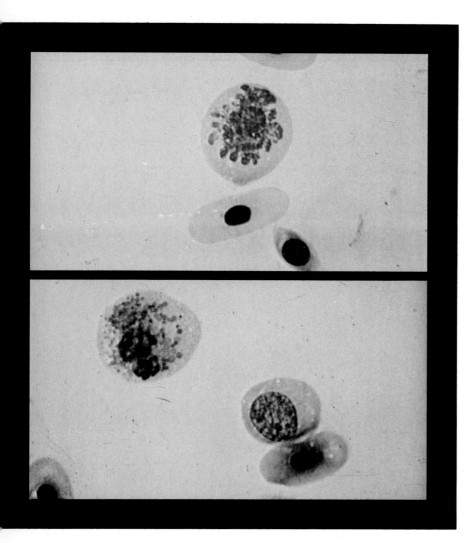

Figures 83a & 83b—Myeloproliferative disease in a turtle.

Figure a: myeloblast in the
prophase; erythrocyte at 6
o'clock position, thrombocyte
at 5 o'clock position.

Figure b: atypical myeloblast.
Both basophilic and eosinophilic granules are present. A
prolymphocyte can be seen
between the myeloblast and
erythrocyte.

Figure 83c—An atypical myeloblast showing pseudo-
podia.

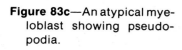

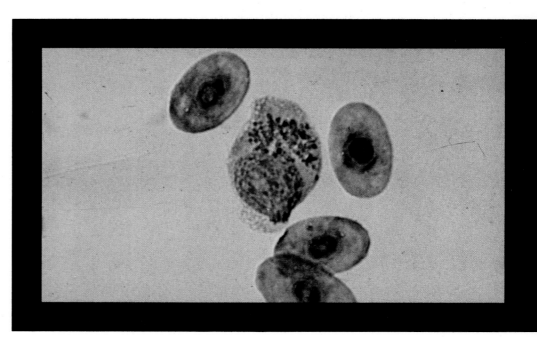

Neoplasia

Figures 83d to 83j
Erythroblasts in a progression of cell divisions.

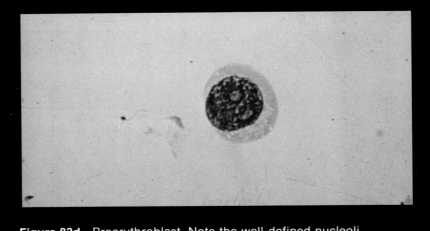

Figure 83d—Proerythroblast. Note the well-defined nucleoli.

Figure 83e—Basophilic erythroblast.   **Figure 83f**—Erythroblast in prophase.

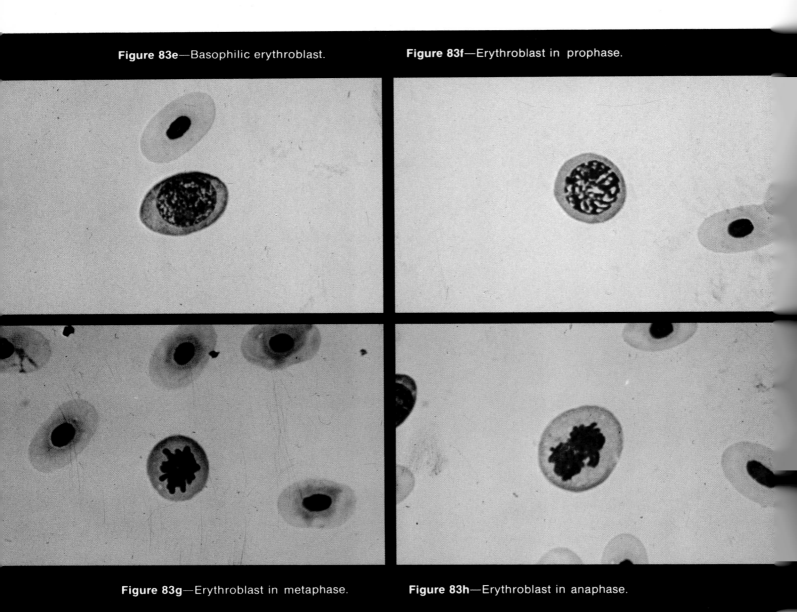

Figure 83g—Erythroblast in metaphase.   **Figure 83h**—Erythroblast in anaphase.

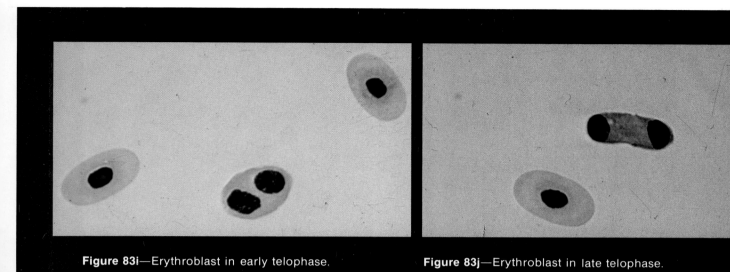

Figure 83i—Erythroblast in early telophase.

Figure 83j—Erythroblast in late telophase.

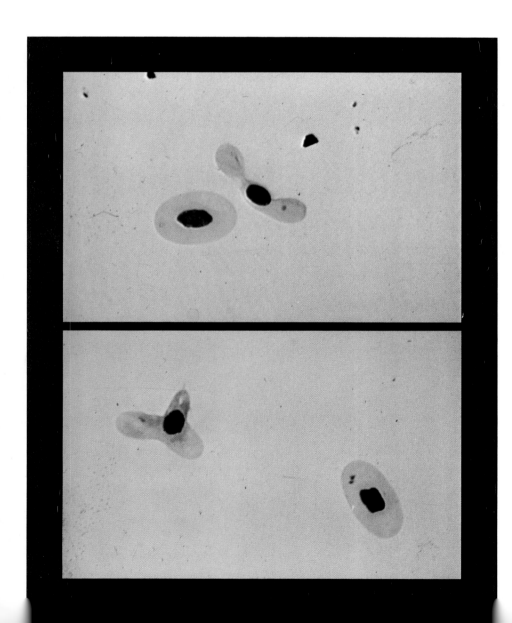

Figure 83k
Atypical erythrocyte.

Figure 83l
Atypical erythrocyte.

Neoplasia

Figures 83m to 83q
Acute lymphatic leukemia
in a boa constrictor.

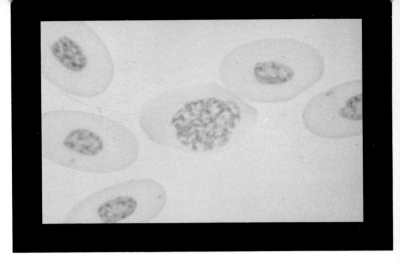

Figure 83m—Lymphoblast in the prophase (x 680).

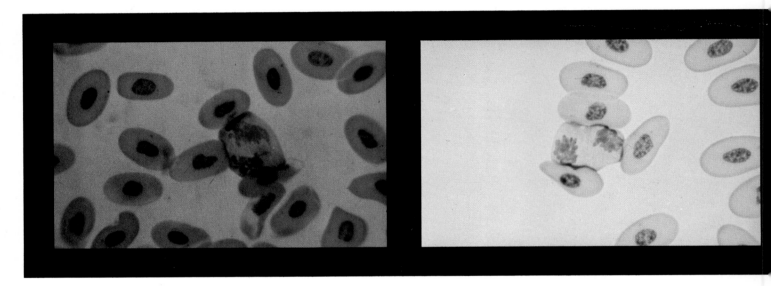

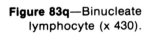—Lymphoblasts in various stages of mitosis.

Figure 83q—Binucleate
lymphocyte (x 430).

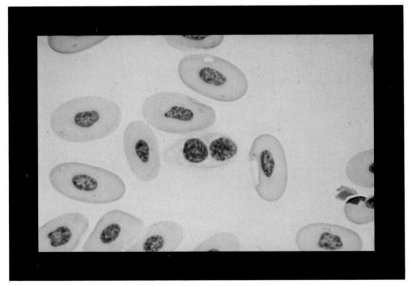

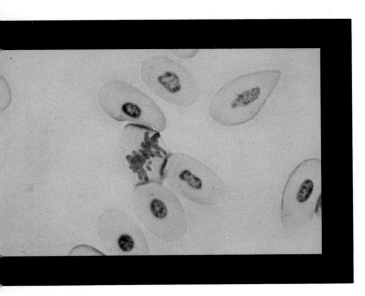

in a boa constrictor (*Figures 83m-83q*). Other interesting tumors were an osteosarcoma in a monitor lizard (*Figures 83r & 83s*), and a fibrosarcoma in a South American boa constrictor (*Figures 83t-83v*).

As more interest is focused on the exotic species, the submission of neoplasms from the lower vertebrates should increase markedly. Perhaps some will serve as models for research into human diseases. A plea has been made for at least a portion of suspected neoplasms (in buffered 10% formalin) to be submitted to:

Registry of Comparative Pathology
Armed Forces Institute of Pathology
Washington, D.C. 20305

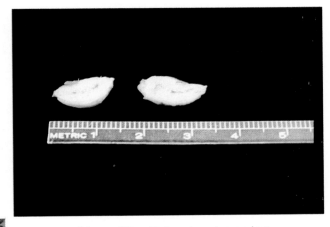

Figure 83r—Osteochondroma in a monitor lizard.

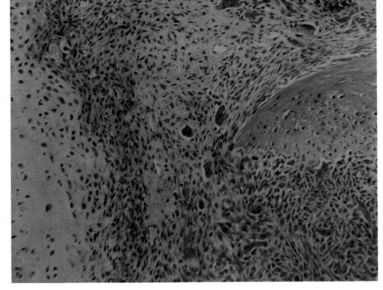

Figure 83s—Histopathologic section of the tumor seen in Figure 83r; sarcoma with osseous and cartilaginous differentiation (H & E x 135). *Photomicrograph courtesy of the Armed Forces Institute of Pathology.*

Figures 83t to 83v—Fibrosarcoma in a boa constrictor.

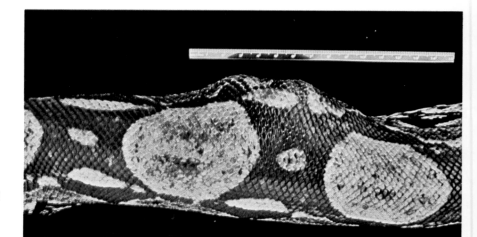

Figure 83t—Gross appearance of the snake prior to surgery.

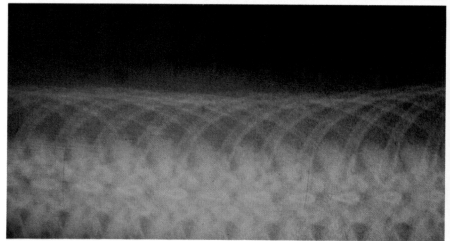

Figure 83u—Postoperative radiograph of the surgical site.

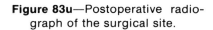
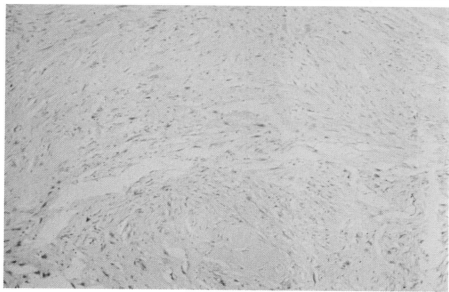

Figure 83v—Histopathologic section. Note the irregular whorls consisting of fibroblasts with collagen interspersed in islands (H & E x 100).

Bibliography

Ashley, L.M.: *Laboratory Anatomy of the Turtle.* Wm. C. Brown Co., Dubuque, Iowa, 1955.

Chiasson, R.B.: *Laboratory Anatomy of the Alligator.* Wm. C. Brown Co., Dubuque, Iowa., 1962.

Dolensek, E.P.: Necropsy Techniques in Reptiles. *JAVMA 159*:1616-1617; 1971.

Frye, F.L.: Surgical Removal of a Cystic Calculus from a Desert Tortoise. *JAVMA 161*:600-602; 1972.

Frye, F.L.: Myeloproliferative Disease in a Turtle. *JAVMA 161*:595-599; 1972.

Frye, F.L.: Blepharoplasty in an Iguana. *VM/SAC 67*: 1110-1111; 1972.

Frye, F.L.; Carney, J.: Acute Lymphatic Leukemia in a Boa Constrictor. *JAVMA* (in press).

Frye, F.L.; Dutra, F.: Fibrosarcoma in a Boa Constrictor, (*Constrictor c., constrictor L.*). *VM/SAC 68*: 245-246; March, 1973.

Gandal, C.P.: A Practical Method of Obtaining Blood from Anesthetized Turtles by Means of a Cardiac Puncture. *Zoologica 43*, Nov. 20, 1958.

Greenfield, L.J.; Morrow, A.G.: The Cardiovascular Hemodynamics of Crocodilia. *J. Surg. Res. 1*:97-103; 1961.

Harris, V.A.: *Anatomy of the Rainbow Lizard.* Hutchinson Tropical Monographs. Hutchinson and Co., London, England, 1963.

Jubb, K.F.V.; Kennedy, P.C.: *Pathology of Domestic Animals.* Academic Press, London, England, 1963; pp. 23-25.

Oldham, J.C.; Smith, H.M.; Miller, S.A.: *A Laboratory Perspectus of Snake Anatomy.* Stipes Publ. Co., Champaign, Ill., 1970.

Page, L.A.: Diseases and Infections of Snakes: A Review. *Bull. Wildlife Dis. Assn.* 2:111-126; 1966.

Schlumberger, H.G.; Lucke, B.: Tumors of Fishes, Amphibians, and Reptiles. *Cancer Res.* 8:657-754; 1948.

Wadsworth, J.R.: Tumors and Tumor-like Lesions of Snakes. *JAVMA 137*:419-420; 1960.

Weickert, C.K.: *Anatomy of the Chordates.* McGraw-Hill Book Co., Inc., New York, N.Y., 1951.

Epilogue

FOR TOO MANY years, organized veterinary medicine has lost — by forfeiture — the practice of captive reptile medicine. The diagnosis and treatment of reptilian disorders traditionally has been left to the zoologists or animal caretakers.

It is my wish that this volume will encourage other veterinarians to explore and find solutions to the myriad clinical entities and practice problems common to the interesting discipline of captive reptile medicine.

As unique findings are made, they should be reported in appropriate publications so that all may share the discoveries.

Glossary

Ambient temperature . . . environmental temperature.

Amniote . . . . any vertebrate that develops an amnion in embryo.

Anurans . . . . the *Salientia,* an order of amphibians including frogs, toads and tree toads.

Birefringent . . . . showing double refraction.

Cachexia . . . . condition of wasting, chronic debility.

Carapace . . . . upper or dorsolateral portion of the shell of a turtle or tortoise.

Chelonia . . . . pertaining to the group of reptiles comprising the turtles, tortoises and terrapins *(Testudinata).*

Crocodilia . . . . pertaining to the group of reptiles comprising the crocodiles, alligators, caimans and gavials.

Dysecdysis . . . . difficult or impaired skin shedding.

Gavial . . . . a large crocodilian differing from other crocodiles by having long, slender jaws with teeth of nearly uniform size; a soft, swollen, inflatable nose tip; and completely webbed feet.

Gynogenesis . . . . development in which the embryo contains only maternal chromosomes following activation of an ovum by sperm that degenerates without fusing with the nucleus of the ovum.

Heterogametic . . . . characterized by the production by one sex of two types of mature germ cells (sperm or ova), one of which produces a male and the other a female.

Hypovitaminosis . . . . condition of insufficiency of one or more vitamins.

Inanition . . . . starvation, multinutritional deficiency.

Melanophore . . . . pigment-containing cell.

Operculum . . . . a body process suggesting a shield or covering flap.

Organoleptic . . . . affecting one or more of the sense organs.

Oviparous . . . . egg-laying.

Ovo-viviparous . . . . birth in which the well-developed progeny are born in eggs, but soon hatch.

Parthenogenesis . . . . reproduction by the development of an egg without its being fertilized by a spermatozoon.

Photoperiod . . . . time interval during which there is significant light energy.

Plastron . . . . ventral portion of the shell of a turtle or tortoise.

Polyspermy . . . . the entrance of more than one sperm into an ovum.

Postprandial . . . . following a meal.

Pseudoneoplasms . . . . . . false tumors; nontumorous masses.

Saurian . . . . pertaining to the group of reptiles comprising the lizards.

Serpentes . . . . pertaining to the group of reptiles comprising the snakes.

Tricholith . . . . gastrointestinal hair (or feather) mass.

Tympanum . . . . ear drum.

Viviparous . . . . live birth.

Index